The knowledge of experience

Dana Mahr

The knowledge of experience

Exploring epistemic diversity in digital
health, participatory medicine,
and environmental research

palgrave
macmillan

Dana Mahr
Faculty of Science
University of Geneva
Geneve, Switzerland

ISBN 978-981-16-3701-8   ISBN 978-981-16-3702-5   (eBook)
https://doi.org/10.1007/978-981-16-3702-5

Cover illustration: Pattern © Melisa Hasan

This Palgrave Macmillan imprint is published by the registered company Springer Nature Singapore Pte Ltd.
The registered company address is: 152 Beach Road, #21-01/04 Gateway East, Singapore 189721, Singapore

Preface

To write this book is both something strange and at the same time very personal. During the research that led to this book, I often felt like an intruder. I rummaged through many feminist archives. I held in my hands original sources of women who reported very intimately about how they perceived their bodies and how they perceived the scientific and political access to this body. I have analysed photos of vaginal self-examinations and read many books about the women's health movement. I have spoken with women from marginalised communities whose reproductive self-determination has been questioned by others. I have interviewed female sex workers who are also makers and diy-biologists trying to involve more women in the decolonisation of their own bodies. And finally, in recent years I have followed, via media and first-person accounts, the social backlash in many Western democracies when it comes to the issue of abortion.

I have dared to do all this although the experience of my own femininity, which for more than thirty years of my life, was not based on physical being but rather on an innate inarticulate inner experience. Some (trans-exclusive) feminists might say that, as a transgender woman, I am not qualified to write about female bodies as much as, perhaps, my cis-gender female partner would be able to do. Nor, they may say, am I qualified to speak about the various forms in which women generate complementary scientific knowledge about these bodies that differs epistemically from the knowledge produced within the classic value framework of science (Green 2006). Although some might argue that I cannot comprehend the full physical experience of being a woman, whether in terms of menstrual cycles, pregnancy, sexuality, or certain forms of social recognition, I find myself on a journey that fundamentally transforms both my private identity and my scientific persona. Perhaps, I can understand my partial outsider status as a transgender person as an epistemic strategy that helps me to better comprehend the connection between epistemic diversity and a more conservative understanding of science. I hope to be respectful on this journey and to contribute to the way in which the female experience and body knowledge intertwine to generate a specific epistemological position. This epistemological position first emerged in the 1970s and has undergone various cycles of transformation since then. It is astonishing to me how deeply experience as practice and reflective theory-building in the field of feminist epistemology are connected and what socio-historical influence this co-genesis had on the diversified field of the women's movement. Simultaneously, as an insider and outsider, I hope to make a small contribution to the expanding corpus of feminist literature written from the perspective of the Science and Technology Studies.

Geneve, Switzerland   Dana Mahr

Contents

List of Figures

1

Introduction

Abstract Why is it important to revisit epistemic diversity in science, technology, and medicine? In the introduction of this book, the author presents her vision for revitalising trust in the institution of science, which is based on integrating individual experiential knowledge from marginalised social groups into the production of epistemic knowledge. Instead of a narrow focus on social representation, the author argues to rethink the practical dimensions of scientific knowledge production themselves.

Keywords Science and society • Citizen science • Open science • Science and democracy

It is winter 2020. I am sitting here in my apartment in Geneva, Switzerland. It is the second or even third wave of the SARS-CoV-2 pandemic that has hit our city pretty hard, and I am socially isolating myself from others. The university where I am employed is closed again and so I work from home. In addition to writing articles, planning conferences, and almost endless meetings via Zoom, I am informed every day about the relevance of my research project. Hidden within the media livestream of "Pandemic-News", in the British Guardian, the New York Times, and the seemingly endless reports of CNN, ABC or the Swiss news channels, is a strange undertone encoded. The experiences of women with the pandemic of 2020 are very different from those of many (but certainly not all) men. There are reports that, in connection with lockdown measures, there has been a significant increase in domestic violence against women (Bradbury-Jones and Isham 2020). Further, the risk of poverty for women (especially of those who are members of minority groups) has increased drastically (Yancy 2020), and women's access to their own bodies is becoming more and more restricted in the face of this crisis (Todd-Gher and Shah 2020). To put it in a nutshell: the coronavirus might become a disaster for feminism in general and the progress of women's health advocacy in particular (Lewis 2020; Wide 2020; Adams 2020; Hollander and Carr 2020).

With many nations under strict stay-at-home orders and several US states like Arkansas, Oklahoma, and Texas suspending access to surgical abortions during the SARS-CoV-2 crisis, the ongoing cultural war about women's reproductive rights has further been intensified (WHO 2020). While conservative Christian groups, so-called "pro-life" advocates and conservative politicians evoke in their recent attacks images of abortion clinics as infectious hotspots and abortion providers as greedy capitalists doing "business as usual" during the pandemic (Paxton 2020), "pro-choice" institutions are promoting telemedical counselling and pharmaceutical abortions as a new solution for desperate women. US programs like "TelAbortion" seek to expand their FDA approved services as fast as possible in order to keep up with a rising tide of demand during the lockdown period. In response to this perceived threat, a Republican senator recently introduced a bill "to prohibit chemical abortions performed without the presence of healthcare providers" (S. 3252). It seems that the next arena of conservative campaigns against Roe vs. Wade (1973) will be the virtual sphere. Despite such attacks, in April 2020 alone, TelAbortion provided well over 800 consultations in the states where the service operates, distributing abortion pills and monitoring their use through zoom meetings and smartphone apps. For Elizabeth Raymond, a senior medical associate at Gynuity Health Projects and leader of the program, the coronavirus crisis might be a litmus test for the democratisation of medical services in the virtual sphere (Belluck 2020). In parallel, TelAbortion uses on its website language reminiscent of the feminist activism, evoking the imagery of women-led online spaces, accessibility, and privacy (TelAbortion 2020) but transferred into a domestic setting. Although this form of telemedicine may be a solution for many involuntarily pregnant individuals, it also creates new problems. One such problem is connected to the fact that involuntary pregnancy is a reality that intersects, for some demographics, with settings of domestic abuse (Braveman 2010). How, one might ask, can telemedicine work when a huge part of one's problem is actually part of the private sphere?

In times of curfews and stay-at-home orders, such questions are shedding light on the challenges for technologically mediated women's health advocacy and medical practice. Neither smartphones nor video conferences are able to replace, in situations of domestic abuse, the refuge of safe-spaces since they lack a design that integrates the individual experience of many women in difficult life situations. This partial blindness to women's experiences by institutional actors concerning abortion in 2020 has also revitalised countercultural approaches and other participatory practices at the grassroots level. Although far from being hostile towards technology, nongovernmental and non-profit feminist groups like WIDE+, the Spanish GynePunk Movement, or the Hesperian Health Guides (Mahr and Prüll 2018), have established during March and April 2020 new infrastructures seeking to blend the 1970s practice of "self-help" with feminist online resources (Baxandall and Gordon 2020). These resources span from participatory open-source information repositories to 3D printable self-help kits for women in social isolation.[1] At the same time, these resources are incorporated into the formation of interpersonal and intercultural support networks, pop-up clinics and illegal underground safe spaces that are, for example, accessible via the Hesperian smartphone app Safe Abortion, feminist WhatsApp groups, or in the analogue form of flyers. In so doing, the respective organisers seek to take the experiences and lifeworlds of women and other minority groups

---

[1] Most prominently is the Mendely group "Gender and COVID-19" initiated by the feminist researcher Rosemary Morgan at Johns Hopkins University (Gender and Covid-19 2020).

during the pandemic seriously. The access to both healthcare and (sub-) culture specific spaces such as community centres, bars, bookstores, and events has become largely limited during the pandemic leaving the vulnerable even more vulnerable (Stern 2020). Therefore, the goal of current activism at the boundaries of physical and mental health for such demographics has adopted a participatory approach that seeks to co-produce knowledge about the impact of COVID-19 on women, migrants, and LGBTQIA+ individuals in more detail, while seeking to find substitutes or new solutions for their lost infrastructures.

This short overview on the health of marginalised social groups during the pandemic of 2020 is not only important for a better understanding of intersectional vulnerabilities in times of crisis, it also sheds light on current trends in the relationship between science and society in general. Keywords for this are *digitalisation*, *democratisation*, and *spatiality* (e.g. domesticity) and their multi-faceted connections. Along this entanglement, I seek to explore in this book what it means both socially and epistemologically to produce scientific knowledge differently in the second decade of the twenty-first century. But what do I mean by *differently* and how can this *differently done science* be related to *more classic approaches towards science*?

In response, some may say: hasn't it become commonplace during the last two decades, that diversity can be of great benefit to science? In June 2018, for example, the editors of *Nature* emphasised that a more diverse workforce within the "hard sciences" could produce new and unimagined insights. For example, white researchers tend to use Caucasian people's tissue and blood for drug testing and therapies for diverse populations, although it is well known that different ethnic groups may have different susceptibilities to disease (Nature 2020). But what is the answer or formula for diversity in science? Would it be to implement new recruitment strategies that consider diverse biographical, identity, and cultural backgrounds? This is already being done (Langford-Hall 2016). Or should we democratise science more? What more could we want from science than open data, open source, open methodology, open peer review, open access, open educational resources, and the possibility to partake in knowledge production beyond classic scientific institutions (Hecker et al. 2018; see Mahr et al. 2018)? Such questions, which resurfaced after many of my lectures at the Universities of Geneva, Bielefeld and Lübeck, I often answered with a counter-question: *What really is the attractiveness of openness and participation, given that the institutional foundations of scientific knowledge production, i.e. its value foundations and power structures, remain unchanged?* Together with my friend and colleague Sascha Dickel, I have shown in an article about "citizen science beyond invited participation" that most participatory research programs of our days adhere to the classic distinction between certified experts and non-certified amateurs, and even goes as far as to cement it. In the digitalised sphere of many citizen science projects, volunteers are assigned the role of data collectors or data analysts, whereby data analysis does not incorporate much freedom or creativity. However, it is more reminiscent of the geometry games for small children, in which differently shaped building blocks have to be inserted into a larger mould with holes of prefabricated shapes (Mahr and Dickel 2019). New methodological or theoretical knowledge coming from outsiders (e.g. the experiential knowledge of marginalised groups that are underrepresented in scientific institutions) is very difficult to develop and utilise in such a framework. Of course, we cannot all suddenly become scientific experts, as the philosopher Harry Collins states in one of his more recent popular science books (Collins 2015). But I think we can at least demand that the polytonality of our positions and experiences be at least represented, heard and taken seriously as a corrective momentum for the proponents of established science. Regardless of the varying viewpoints, the problem of a lack of diversity is not only one of representation, socio-economic background, or organisation but, so the main thesis of this book, epistemic in nature. Nevertheless, current democratisation policies seem to be blind to this problem, hence they remain *epistemically conservative*.

The first part of the book is therefore conceptualised as a sociological and historical exploration. This inquiry is based on four questions: What do I mean when I speak of *epistemic conservatism*? What are the social and philosophical conditions that have led mainstream science to resist the diversification of its own foundations? Have groups and individuals already existed, which tried to *do science differently*? If so, how did they imagine both form and practice of science and why haven't they succeeded in their quest for epistemic diversity? Then, within the main chapters of the book I explore what I mean by epistemic diversity in more detail. I understand epistemic diversity as an institutionalised openness to ways of knowledge production that are complementary to classical scientific values and methods and that emerge from the needs of affected social groups. The first case study uses the example of popular online health networks to analyse to what extent the rapid evolution of the digitalisation of our health behaviour demands a new epistemology of the self; one which is based less on narrative creation of meaning but rather one which atomises the individual into a stream of (voluntarily donated) data. This new epistemology of identity, as I will show, has the character of "Silicon Valley Capitalism" and plays with the mistrust in institutions that many of us might feel in order to achieve its goal. At the same time, I will also show, in the case study, to what extent users of such networks are increasingly developing a form of agency that I call digital resilience, rediscovering an intersectional feminist understanding of body knowledge. The second case study focuses on how, in the early twenty-first century, both the social and body-related practices and the theories of the women's health movement of the 1970s are being rediscovered in a new form and by new actors. Vaginal self-examination and menstrual extraction are not only tools for "decolonizing female bodies" (i.e. the reintegration of the female perspective in the production of knowledge), but also *performative practices that seek to expand the limits of what we understand as scientific knowledge*, in both online health networks and in radical feminist groups such as the GynePunks from Barcelona. The third case study explores the distinctly locally oriented epistemology of "Thai Baan" research in the Mekong Delta. In contrast to the "participatory action research" of the 1980s and 1990s, whose topics focused on the needs of people in developing countries often utilising a decidedly Western understanding of knowledge, "village research" in Thailand and Myanmar seeks to find its own ways. We often assumed that local knowledge is somehow different than "proper" scientific knowledge, and that knowledge can only be credible once it has been verified by professional scientists or "the scientific method". While there are differences between local and scientific knowledge, there are also important similarities and pathways to a fruitful interconnection. Like scientific knowledge, local knowledge involves empirical methods, gathering information, analysis and interpretation.

However, local knowledge might be more holistic since it is based on wider sets of experience. This kind of knowledge could give us all an example of how we could overcome the climate crisis. In the last chapter of the book I ask, how science could reinvent itself after what many consider the anti-scientific and anti-diversity backlash of the Trump era. Will we as scientists and scholars be able to pave the way for new and integrative forms of production of scientific knowledge, after this experience? How can we revitalise the institution of science beyond the some of the more problematic legacies of *Western epistemology*?

References

Adams, Patrick. 2020. Amid Covid-19, a Call for M.D.s or Mail the Abortion Pill. *The New York Times* (online). https://www.nytimes.com/2020/05/12/opinion/covid-abortion-pill.html. Visited 25 May 2020. https://doi.org/10.1098/rstb.2013.0152

Baxandall, Rosalyn, and Linda Gordon. 2020. *Dear Sisters. Dispatches form the Women's Liberation Movement*. New York: Basic Books.

Belluck, Pam. 2020. Abortion by Telemedicine: A Growing Option as Access to Clinics Wanes. *The Guardian* (online). https://www.nytimes.com/2020/04/28/health/telabortion-abortion-telemedicine.html?referringSource=articleShare. Accessed 26 May 2020.

Bradbury-Jones, Caroline, and Louise Isham. 2020. The Pandemic Paradox: The Consequences of COVID-19 on Domestic Violence. *Journal of Clinical Nursing. Early View*. https://doi.org/10.1111/jocn.15296.

Braveman, Paula. 2010. Social Conditions, Health Equity, and Human Rights. *Health Human Rights* 12 (2): 31–48. PMID: 21178188.

Collins, Harry. 2015. *Are We All Scientific Experts Now?* Boston: Polity Press.

Gender and Covid-19. 2020. *Open Mendely Group Initiated by Rosemary Morgan*. https://www.mendeley.com/community/gender-and-covid-19/. Accessed 9 Dec 2020.

Hecker, Susanne, Rick Bonney, Muki Haklay, and Franz Hölker, eds. 2018. Innovation in Citizen Science – Perspectives on Science-Policy Advances. *Citizen Science: Theory and Practice* 3 (1). https://doi.org/10.5334/cstp.114. Accessed 9 Dec 2020.

Hollander, Judd E., and Brendan G. Carr. 2020. Virtually Perfect? Telemedicine for Covid-19. *The New England Journal of Medicine* 382: 1679–1681. https://doi.org/10.1056/NEJMp2003539.

Langford-Hall, Mary. 2016. Recruitment, Retention and Mentoring of Minorities into the Fields of Communication Sciences and Disorders. *International Journal of Humanities and Social Science Review* 2 (9): 1–4.

Lewis, Helen. 2020. The Coronavirus Is a Disaster for Feminism. Pandemics Affect Men and Women Differently. *The Atlantic* (online). https://www.theatlantic.com/international/archive/2020/03/feminism-womens-rights-coronavirus-covid19/608302/. Accessed 18 Dec 2020.

Mahr, Dana, and Livia Prüll. 2018. Körperliche Selbstermächtigung aus dem 3D-Drucker? Feministische Kulturen als Parallelwelten und der Kampf um gesellschaftliche Teilhabe seit 1970. In *Kybernetik, Kapitalismus, Revolutionen. Emanzipatorische Perspektiven im technologischen Wandel*, ed. Paul Buckermann, Anne Koppenburg, and Simon Schaub, 161–190. Münster: Unrast.

Mahr, Dana, and Sascha Dickel. 2019. Citizen Science Beyond Invited Participation: Nineteenth Century Amateur Naturalists, Epistemic Autonomy, and Big Data Approaches Avant La Lettre. *History and Philosophy of the Life Sciences* 41 (4). https://doi.org/10.1007/s40656-019-0280-z.

Mahr, Dana, Claudia Göbel, Alan Irwin, and Katrin Vohland. 2018. Watching or Being Watched – Enhancing Productive Discussion Between the Citizen Sciences, the Social Sciences and the Humanities. In *Citizen Science: Innovation in Open Science, Society and Policy*, ed. Susanne Hecker, Muki Haklay, Anne Bowser, Zen Makuch, and Johannes Vogel. London: UCL Press. https://doi.org/10.14324.

Nature. editorial board. anonymous. 2020. Science Benefits from Diversity. Improving he Participation of Under – Represented Groups Is Not Just Fairer – It Could Produce Better Research. *Nature* 558. https://www.nature.com/articles/d41586-018-05326-3. Accessed 18 Dec 2020.

Paxton, Ken. 2020. *Health Care Professionals and Facilities, Including Abortion Providers, Must Immediately Stop All Medically Unnecessary Surgeries and Procedures to Preserve Resources to Fight COVID-19 Pandemic*. https://www.texasattorneygeneral.gov/news/releases/health-care-professionals-and-facilities-including-abortion-providers-must-immediately-stop-all. Accessed 18 Dec 2020.

Roe v. Wade. 410 U.S. 113. 1973. Braveman, Paula. 2010. Social Conditions, *Health Equity, and Human Rights*. *Health Hum Rights* 12 (2): 31–48. PMID: 21178188.

Stern, Jessica. 2020. The Concept of "Safe Spaces" Under COVID-19. *womensnews.org*. https://womensenews.org/2020/05/the-concept-of-safe-spaces-under-covid-19/. Accessed 18 Dec 2020.

TelAbortion. 2020. *Safe. Effective. Private. Convenient.* https://telabortion.org/. Accessed 18 Dec 2020.

Todd-Gher, Jaime, and Payal K. Shah. 2020. Abortion in the Context of COVID-19: A Human Rights Imperative. *Sexual and Reproductive Health Matters* 28 (1). https://doi.org/10.1080/26410397.2020.1758394.

Wide. Feminists transforming Economic Development. 2020. *Covid-19 Crisis from a Feminist Perspective*. https://wideplus.org/2020/03/26/covid-19-crisis-from-a-feminist-perspective-overview-of-different-articles-published/. Accessed 18 Dec 2020.

World Health Organization, WHO. 2020. Q&A: *Violence Against Women During COVID-19.* https://www.who.int/emergencies/diseases/novel-coronavirus-2019/question-and-answers-hub/q-a-detail/violence-against-women-during-covid-19?gclid=Cj0KCQjwupD4BRD4ARIsABJ MmZ-q4EN7Vp4nhEZf7wzAd_VGpIiYzv8o_rAbVdkGzlWb-vK4SZA37apgaAoeaEALw_wcB. Accessed 18 Dec 2020.

Yancy, Clyde W. 2020. COVID-19 and African Americans. *JAMA* 323 (19): 1891–1892. https://doi.org/10.1001/jama.2020.6548. Accessed 18 Dec 2020.

2

Why Is Science the Way It Is Today?

Abstract This chapter asks why, on the one hand, science and technology are more successful than ever and permeate all areas of life, but why, at the same time, more and more people are losing confidence in science and technology. One answer is that both scientific training and popularisation have epistemically conservative foundations that correlate with naïve empiricism. This results in a situation where the inner complexity of scientific knowledge production is obscured. Revisiting epistemic diversity, especially the experiential knowledge of emergent concerned groups, might hold the key for a new, more inclusive, and participatory science for the twenty-first century.

Keywords Epistemic diversity • Epistemic conservatism • Public understanding of science • Experiential knowledge

"Good science" is apolitical, free of individual interests, it is objective, it reveals disembodied true facts, and of course it is "not interested in your feelings" (Shapiro 2019). This image of science is not only represented by young and edgy Harvard graduates, who some media call "conservative

© The Author(s), under exclusive license to Springer Nature Singapore Pte Ltd. 2021
D. Mahr, *The knowledge of experience*, https://doi.org/10.1007/978-981-16-3702-5_2

gladiators" or "cool kid's philosophers" (Tavernise 2017), but it is still also prevalent in public discourse, in parts of the educational system and is even perpetuated (probably also believed in) by some professional scientists. But can science without perspective really be good or even be possible?

There is no doubt that science and technology have greatly enriched humanity over the past two centuries. We can fly around the world, we can communicate instantly with other people using telecommunication technologies, we have made incredible progress in modern medicine, we are exploring the quantum-physical fabric of our reality and we are gaining more and more knowledge about the universe itself. At the same time, however, it is equally true that our technology and our science are also responsible for the horrors of the atomic bomb, for the increasingly rapid change in the planet's climate, for environmental pollution, oil spills, for the profits of both the pharmaceutical industry and the military-industrial complex, as well as growing inequities around the globe. "But wait a moment", some may say, "is it not the social, military, or economic application of science and technology that causes such problems? Scientific knowledge in itself is pure. It is the human factor that makes it impure".

Yet, such a separation of scientific knowledge and its practice is, in my opinion, no more than a *fig leaf*. Scientific knowledge cannot be considered separately from the social conditions of its production. It is both socially and historically determined. Our ideas about what objectivity is and where we find it, for example, are subject to temporal factors, as historian Lorraine Daston and sociologist Peter Galison have pointed out in their book Objectivity (2010). In eighteenth century natural history, idealistic philosophy determined what was objective. Truly real objects could only be found in the divine imagination. For example, the theoretical symmetry of the plants and animals depicted in atlases was considered more true than actual specimens. The "mechanical objectivity" of the late nineteenth and early twentieth century aimed at eliminating the universal human tendency of valuation and aesthetisation. The cold gaze of the newly invented camera was thus elevated to a medium of objectivity. In the late twentieth century, however, rose the tendency to understand the technical image not as objective per se. The image itself, which was now only perceived as a representation of reality, had no meaning. It needed a translator again. Now trained observers (e.g. medical experts), who could draw meaning from the representations and models, became carriers of objectivity (Daston 2001).

Such examples illuminate the fact that objectivity is made by humans who are situated temporally, politically, socially, sexually and along the lines of many other factors. Their biases and preferences implicitly determine the produced knowledge, both in "hard" and "soft" fields of enquiry. This "situatedness of objectivity" also concerns apparently completely neutral entities of knowledge, such as algorithms (Pasquale 2015). When Apple integrated FaceID into its iOS smartphone operating system in 2018, the first few weeks saw many users who were people of colour (or women) excluded from their devices. Internal analysis by Apple finally revealed that the algorithm used was not sufficiently trained to recognise the faces of women or people of colour, because the predominantly white and male programmers had simply used people who looked like themselves as a benchmark for the training of the programme. This was not a bad intention but rather an unconscious bias, as we can find it in medical or epidemiological research. To refer to a book by the historian and sociologist of science Steven Shapin, science is "never pure" (2010). But if this is the case, why do so many people still believe in the disembodied objectivity of science? Why do some people even call for an epistemic cultural war to defend this form of objectivism against perspectivism in science? This chapter tries to find an answer to these questions.

2.1   Epistemic Conservatism

"Grab 'em by the facts" This slogan, which I encountered for the first time in April 2017 on the March for Science in Geneva (Switzerland) still intrigues me today. This sentence summaries, in an almost epitomic way, the socio-cultural situation at the intersection of politics, society, science, and truth that has preoccupied many of us since the beginning of the Trump presidency. The dripping misogyny of Donald J. Trump, revealed in the leaked "Access Hollywood" recordings from 2005, is ironically paired with the eclectic attitude of his administration towards scientific knowledge, especially when it comes to human-made climate change and questions surrounding gender and sex. Kellyanne Conway's neologism "alternative facts" had just caused confusion and concern in the scientific community in January of said year and the ironic reversal and integration of Trump's verbal blunder into a protest slogan therefore had a certain political "punch". Even in 2019, I still occasionally saw cars that have this slogan as bumper stickers, both in the US and Europe.

But when I read the protester's slogan today in midst of the Covid19 crisis, it makes me think about it in a different way and I recognise that there might be something slightly (but nevertheless dangerously) off with the ideal it seems to promote: facts are laws of nature set in stone. They are cold, neutral, and absolute. It's an idea of science that, unfortunately, plays more into the hands of social divisions and alienation of large sections of the public from science rather than fostering productive engagement. Is it possible to counter the self-referential eclecticism that has been the driving force behind Trump's science policy with scholastic epistemic materialism? I think not, since both ways of understanding science and scientific facts are fundamentally flawed and more closely connected than one might think. This is particularly evident when facts are "made hard" (what a phallic picture) to generate political or discursive authority. For example, the alt-right figurehead and conservative political commentator Ben Shapiro, during his attacks on feminist issues, can claim that "facts don't care about your feelings" and thus utilise (or even embody) a similar epistemic position as the young female pro-science demonstrator with her protest sign. Yet, from an epistemological point of view, facts are neither arbitrary nor absolute but simultaneously material and constructed.

2.2   What Are Scientific Facts?

In the same year that I participated in the "March for Science" the philosopher of science Christoper ChoGlueck wrote a very accessible and poignant post on the SciU blog of Indiana University clarifying the characteristics of scientific facts. He starts by presenting a simple (but highly politicised) scientific fact: *The Earth's atmosphere has warmed in recent decades in an unexpected and unforeseen way.* This statement, which is based on an IPCC report from 2014 (IPCC 2014), has no explanatory value in the sense of causation, but rather is a statement of fact. But where, ChoGlueck asks, in what is the factual and scientific character of the statement grounded (ChoGlueck 2017)?

First of all, it is an *empirical statement*, which includes experiences with the world and not just reasoning based on logic and theory. In our every-day lives, we experience for example the weather of the city or town we are living in and then categorise it along traditional categories such as rainy, cold, warm, cloudy, sunny, and so forth. We are even able to his-toricise those first-hand experiences and transform them into statements like "In my childhood we always had snow at Christmas". Yet such dec-larations remain anecdotal and individual, at least when we apply classi-cal epistemological categories. Most of us are not actually keeping journals with weather charts and temperature measurements. And, even if we would do so, we still would not be able to make any assertions about global scale climate change. Let us assert, for the sake of argument, that my family has kept records about the weather of our home town for the last 100 years. How could we argue for a general trend against the back-drop of such spatially limited information? What value would our diary of information even have on a larger scale? And even if we could compare our information with the information of many other collectors, how could we be sure that we all measured in the same way, under similar conditions, with compatible categories, and instruments? The produc-tion of scientific facts about "the climate" or other large phenomena depend not only on empirical information but also on *community* and a shared understanding of what to observe, how this observation is done, and a shared set of rules for "good observational" practice. As ChoGlueck writes in his blog post, "scientists don't work in isolation but in commu-nities, exchanging and critiquing each other's findings and ideas" (Ibid). A scientific fact in the field of climate science is therefore not derived from only one set of observations "but from countless collections from all over the world" (Ibid), which also extend temporarily. But very much like the climate the categories and standards of the scientific community are also changing over time. For this reason, NASA climate scientists have marked the year 1880 as the start of modern global record keeping. Their rationale for this distinction: earlier available climate information doesn't cover enough the earth geographically to supply accurate readings for twenty-first century standards and computational purposes. This is because they are often not transmitted in a quantified (or at least quantifiable) form, which could be utilised as data for modern models of climate development. Scientific facts are neither merely given natural entities, nor are they just mere constructions of the human mind. They are rather an amalgam of empirical, methodical, technological, social, spatial, and historical factors. This is because the world around us may be given, but we can only make sense of the entities in it by cognitive distinctions, which must be significant for us. And since we as Homo Sapiens are social primates, these meaningful differentiation processes are of intersubjective nature.

This social side of facts was first described by the Polish physician and biologist Ludwik Fleck in the 1930s. In his monograph "Entstehung und Entwicklung einer wissenschaftlichen Tatsache" (Engl.: "Origin and Development of a Scientific Fact") published in 1935, he analysed that scientific facts are both historical and socially constructed (Fleck 2017 (=1935)). As a case study for this, he used the facticity of the relation between the so-called "Bordet-Wassermann reaction" and syphilis (Ibid: p. 2). He shows that both traditional descriptions of this disease as "Lustseuche" ("plague of lust") or (with racist undertones) "Franzosenkrankheit" ("morbus gallicus" = French disease) and contemporary shifts in the understanding of immunology intermingled in how the scientific community produced facts about this plague of the *fin de siècle*. Neither the French researchers Jules Bordet and Otave Gengou, who five years prior developed the serological complement fixation test, nor Paul von Wassermann and Julius Citron who finally developed a first working syphilis test at the Robert Koch Institute for Infectious Diseases in 1906 "discovered" their facts independently from pre-exiting "thinking styles" ("Denkstile"). The contemporary, but no less misogynistic, idea that syphilis was essentially transmitted by women who prostitute themselves was coupled in their writings and essays with the burgeoning idea that the human immune system might function similarly to a strict police that keeps unwanted individuals from the streets (Ehrlich and Gonder 1914).

Such ideas not only pre-determined how Wassermann and his colleagues shaped syphilis as a research object but also their choice of epistemological tools such as test designs, equipment, and selection of human test subjects like pregnant women for antibody studies. While proponents of the logical positivism, such as the Vienna Circle, postulated the possibility that scientists could adopt a neutral and objective position towards their research objects (Uebel 2020), Flecks' analysis of the intertwined paths, pre-existing ideas, and assumptions that co-produced the factual link between the "Bordet-Wassermann reaction" and the syphilis showed that a scientific description of the world is closely linked to the pre-scientific experience of and socially internalised assumptions about the world. In his own words:

> A truly isolated investigator is impossible (…). An isolated investigator without bias and tradition, without forces of mental society acting upon him, and without the effect of the evolution of that society, would be blind and thoughtless. Thinking is a collective activity (…). Its product is a certain picture, which is visible only to anybody who takes part in this social activity, or a thought which is also clear to the members of the collective only. What we do think and how we do see depends on the thought-collective to which we belong. (Fleck 2017 (=1935))

Accordingly, Fleck proposed the sociological and historical reconstruction of the genesis of accepted scientific facts as a medium for scientific development. The reflection and relativisation of common dogmas in methods and theories, as well as the constant re-evaluation of what the scientific community understands as facts, should thus, according to Fleck, become an intrinsic practice of scientific endeavours. Although this sociological approach to epistemology was initially ill received by his contemporaries, it became a basic building block in the formation of the science and technology studies a few decades later. Thus, Thomas Kuhn developed his concept of scientific paradigms, which represent the historical-sociologically determined (presupposed and unquestioned) doctrines of a discipline, from that of the "thinking style". Recent research devoted to the historicisation of epistemology is also rooted in Fleck's work (Daston 2001; Daston and Galison 2010).

2.3   PUS: Problematic Understanding of Science

Even though the hybrid character of facts, as both given in the world and socially determined, has long become commonplace among scholars of the science and technology studies and many practicing scientists, the public image of scientific facts remains predominantly objectivistic (Weingart 2001). There are many reasons for this, of which I will mention only two here. Firstly, in public discourse science is often reduced to its systemic function as a "truth generator" (Mahr and Dickel 2019). Paradoxically, this perception has led to a loss of trust in the course of the politicisation and economisation of scientific knowledge in recent decades. Experts contradict each other publicly on television and spectacular cases of problematic industry-financed research, such as that of the tobacco industry, have been uncovered (Boyle et al. 2010; Marshall 1987). Even if many people recognise scientists as fallible people because of this, they still fall back on the idea that the *scientific method* can in itself generate value-free and objective facts. In the perception of such actors, it is not the institution of science that inserts values or certain interests into research, but the human factor. The finding that values and interests are part of the epistemic foundations of scientific knowledge production is often ignored.

Secondly, some popular science popularisers are portraying science as an institution that is under constant attack by pseudo-scientific systems of thought such as homeopathy, the denial of human-made climate change, or creationism in its new form of Intelligent Design. Individuals, like the palaeontologist Stephen Jay Gould or the evolutionary biologist Richard Dawkins, present themselves to the public as fighters and saviours of science. They reject the findings of the sociology of science and other fields of the STS as relativistic. Such relativism would, so they argue, ultimately enable fringe groups and pseudo-scientists to challenge "proper" science as "just a theory". In a blog-post from 2015 Dawkins, for example, states "Philosophers, I am aware, can be relied upon to cloud even the word fact" (Dawkins 2015). Instead of following philosophers, scientists and science popularisers should rather begin to use the term in its (objectivist) every-day definition: "Courts of law, newspapers, and all of us in everyday life use the word fact in a way that few have difficulty in understanding. It is a fact that New Zealand is in the Southern Hemisphere (Barack Obama is a US President, it is now raining in Oxford, grass is green etc.). It is this everyday usage of fact that we should be concerned with when we advocate evolution to lay audiences (Ibid)". Thus, he not only draws a strangely anachronistic picture of a rather incompetent public but also suggests the disguising of the way scientists and science as an institution actually work. Even if creationists and other pseudo-scientific movements would indeed pose a threat to the scientific education of future generations, I consider the actions of Dawkins and his comrades-in-arms to be highly problematic. Through the reach of their publications and media appearances, however, their position currently seems to fall on fertile ground. The demonstrator I met in 2017 seems to have based her protest sign at least on such kind of concept of facts.

Figures like Dawkins, however, do not limit their demarcation activities only to social phenomena such as modern creationism, but increasingly extends it to widely agreed upon sub-areas of the humanities and social sciences. The prominent German plant physiologist Ulrich Kutschera, for example, recently caused a controversy with harsh biologistic attacks on the achievements of the gender studies. In their differentiation between biological sex and social gender, the gender studies would, so he stated, completely negate the evolutionary-biological foundations of human societies. Characteristics and behaviours described as classically male and classically female would be inscribed deeply into us genetically. In his book "The Gender Paradox. Man and woman as evolved human types" ("German: Das Gender Paradoxon. Mann und Frau als evolvierte Menschentypen") he portrays scholars like Judith Butler, who emphasise the performativity of gender, as radical-feminist ideologists that appropriate biological terms to impose their political agenda (Kutschera 2018). In his view, gender mainstreaming in particular represents a "woman-equal-man ideology" based on the "false teachings" of the American psychologist John Money (1921–2006). Kutschera claims that it is a proven fact that most differences between man and woman, including certain behaviours, are ultimately based on the chromosome sets XY and XX (Ibid).

Over the past two decades, such claims have been discredited not only by social scientists but also by other biologists, medical experts and other representatives of the STEM sciences. Exemplary for this development is a new approach in the cognitive neurosciences. During the 1990s and 2000s, most neuroscientists embraced the then new technology of magnetic resonance imaging. This technology promised to fulfil the dream, cherished for more than a century in their thought collective, of precisely localising the function of the human brain. A gold-digger mood flared up in their field of research, which silenced critical voices that had been wary of a technologically induced revival of phrenology. Only after an unmanageable amount of data had been collected, which ultimately proved to be inconsistent and contradictory, did the first researchers begin to question the paradigm of MRI localisation. The recorded brain activities proved to be too erratic. Networks of electrical impulses appeared and died out. When researchers thought they had located something significant, the electrical impulses escaped their mapping and reappeared, apparently without reason, in completely different regions of the brain. As in the early twentieth century, the object of their research once more eluded their understanding. Gradually, however, a new paradigm began to emerge in the thinking of neuroscientists: plasticity (Alvarez-Salvado et al. 2014).

According to scientists like Marco Taubert and his team at the Max Planck Institute for Human Cognitive and Brain Sciences, "we never use the same brain twice". The new keyword in the neurosciences, the new fact, is emergent plasticity (Taubert et al. 2012). Various neurological processes emerge in ever-changing brain areas, thus making older notions that, for example, a very specific location for emotions, language or logic, exist obsolete. Hence, social imprinting is given greater scope. Cases such as that of William Buttars, a normally developed boy, missing one half of his brain since birth, can be better explained in this new paradigm and the fact of plasticity (Rubino 2015). This new paradigm had a ripple effect. Therefore, also other claims associated with the old idea of a brain atlas no longer fit into our altered picture of human cognition, including what the neuroscientist Gina Rippon, a researcher at the Aston Brain Center in Birmingham, describes as "neurosexism" (2019). Against the background of plasticity the human brain turns out to be an organ that is structured and restructured essentially through the experiences of an individual. Male and female brains, therefore exist in a mostly reactive form, shaping and structuring themselves around how our social environment frames us, what we experience and what we learn from others. A gendered brain isn't given, it is, to use a quote by Simone de Beauvoir in a very loosely way, made.

Accordingly, when feminist theorists like Judith Butler describe gender as performative, their theories are ultimately more compatible with current scientific knowledge than Kutschera's interpretations of human evolution, physiology and behaviour as largely pre-determined. Sexual differentiation of human brains thus shifted its "facticity" into a more socially determined direction. Therefore, the simple association of brain developments and gendered behaviours with XY and XX chromosomes is fading into the annals of the history of science. Facts are not simply there, rather, we derive them from nature, evaluate them against the background of individual and societal norms and believes. All in an attempt to make sense of the world.

Another example to illustrate the complexity and perspectivity of scientific facts is my own journey and the ontological status of my identity. In the reductionist viewpoint of Kutschera and many other "gender-critical" authors, I might be just a funny little man that pretends to be a women. Contrary to this claim, the overwhelming consensus of contemporary research in developmental biology shows that social and biological reality find their expression in interacting layers. The findings of the field of systems medicine, which explores the interplay of genome, epigenome, proteome, metabolome, microbiome and social influences on human individuals is instructive for this viewpoint (see Roukos 2012). Against this backdrop, the gender I was assigned at birth is more difficult to recognise than a biologistic and reductive viewpoint might suggest. I have feminine facial features, no beard, I behave quite normally like any other woman. If one were to try to question my femininity with "scientific methods", then behavioural studies and an external examination of my body would not be conclusive. But, one may ask, what about internal tests, a hormonal blood test for example. Such findings would not be conclusive either, since (at least in light of my last endocrinological findings from January 2020) the composition of my sexual hormones (estrogen, progesterone, and testosterone) is like (as result of a hormonal replacement therapy) that of a cis-gender woman (who associates herself with the sex attributed to her at birth). Hence, even on this level my body would be categorised as female by the vast majority of observers and analysts. But what about other characteristics, such as my primary sexual organs some might ask? Apart from the fact that you should never ask anyone what they have in their pants, it is almost certain that I do not have ovaries and a womb. But, this is also true for many other women, whether from birth or in the course of a hysterectomy due to a disease or an accident. What about a genetic test? Isn't this in Kutschera's eyes the one decisive criterium? I, as well as all my doctors, do not know the setup of my chromosomes. I never had a corresponding genetic test, which, by the way, might also apply to the majority of the world's population. Although I am quite sure that I am born with XY chromosomes, the significance of chromosomes is not as indisputable for sex determination as some would like it to be.

The genomic resource centre of the World Health Organization (WHO) clarifies the variety of human gender expressions on its homepage like following:

> Humans are born with 46 chromosomes in 23 pairs. The X and Y chromosomes determine a person's sex. Most women are 46XX and most men are 46XY. Research suggests, however, that in a few births per thousand some individuals will be born with a single sex chromosome (45X or 45Y) (sex monosomies) and some with three or more sex chromosomes (47XXX, 47XYY or 47XXY, etc.) (sex polysomies). In addition, some males are born 46XX due to the translocation of a tiny section of the sex determining region of the Y chromosome. Similarly some females are also born 46XY due to mutations in the Y chromosome. Clearly, there are not only females who are XX and males who are XY, but rather, there is a range of chromosome complements, hormone balances, and phenotypic variations that determine sex. (WHO 2015)

Given this knowledge, the categorisation of intersex and other individuals with differing sexual characteristics (and identities) into binary categories reveals itself as problematic. Their existence is not a birth defect, like some conservative commoners might argue, but rather the expression of a normal variation of phenotypic expressions within the human species (Viloria and Nieto 2020). Representative studies by biologist and gender researcher Anne Fausto-Sterling have shown that more than one percent of the world's population might be born with sex anatomy variations that deviate from binary categories (Fausto-Sterling 1993, 2012; Fausto-Sterling and Stein 2004). Such variations might be visible ambiguous sexual characteristics or subtle genetic differences, as regarded in above mentioned WHO statement.

In recent years, the acceptance of differences in gender and sexual diversity has become increasingly visible. Surgical and hormonal interventions to assign a binary gender to newborns have been challenged by bioethicists and intersex activists (von Wahl 2019). Both many people on the intersex spectrum, as well as those of us who define themselves as transgender, demand social visibility and participation (Carpenter 2018). These are, among others, the Vogue supermodel Hanne Gaby Odiele, the Jamaican-born British writer Lady Colin Campbell, the South African gold-medalist runner Caster Semenya, and the British actress and "Bond-Girl" Caroline Cossesy. Yet also, and more importantly, the countless individuals who are not celebrities but nevertheless rise up to be accepted by society (Magubane 2014). I hope that these examples clarified that the fact of gender and sex cannot be reduced into the binary of XY and XX chromosomes. Rather, the facticity of gender and sex is expressed on different ontological levels of an individual's existence. Appearance, behaviour, endocrinology, epigenetic expressions, or our genetic setup represent themselves as facts, yet their facticity is not only bound to human observation but also lived experience. The decision about which ontological level we choose to describe or someone else's gender is ultimately social.

Most of us avoid complexity, in our everyday lives and (if we work in this field) in scientific contexts. We reduce it in our models, for example of climate change, in order to be able to make statements at all. We are psychologically primed to be solution-focused. We don't like it when we can't explain something easily, and our political systems are based on making simple choices between political action A or B. Influential philosophers of science have even elevated "simplicity" to an "intrinsic value" of science (Daston 2001). Complexity reduction is also a determining factor in the educational system. Of course, scientific facts are taught in a very reduced and simplified form. The many ambivalences and ambiguities that exist in the reality of scientific enquiry are not highlighted in most curricula. But such reductions also make us vulnerable in other respects. The invocation of facts can become a weapon, especially when the epistemic, social, and discursive functions of facts, which are on ontological different levels, are merged to achieve a specific (oftentimes political) goal. In the case of trans-exclusionary feminism certain forms of institutionalised knowledge, like the role of chromosomes for the development of human bodies, become de-contextualised and discursively utilised to disqualify facts that exist on another ontological level, like the existence of transgender individuals in our societies (Mahr and Prüll 2018).

Beyond the sensitivities of epistemically reductionist popularisers or those of political authors like Shapiro or J.K. Rowling and the conservative YouTube channel PragerU, new educational formats appear which address the complexity of scientific knowledge and the variability of facts. One example of the latter is Bill Nye's new Netflix show "Bill Nye Saves the World" first aired in 2017. In the episode "The Sexual Spectrum", for example, he explains how transgender identity emerges on an epigenetic level during pregnancy and emphasises the naturalness and normality of intersex individuals by utilising participatory and illustrative methods. In addition, a new generation of science popularisers rises. Prominent YouTubers such as Mai Thi Nguyen-Kim (@maithi_NK), Abigail Thorn (@PhilosophyTube), Natalie Wynn (@ContraPoints) or Harris Michael "Harry" Brewis (@Hbomberguy) take the complexity of scientific knowledge as the subject of their video essays. In contrast to the previous generation of popularisers, they do not shy away from the uncomfortable, uncertain and provisional nature scientific knowledge. Their success shows that at least some parts of the public in the twenty-first century are not afraid to understand science as something deeply human.

2.4   Lost Trust and the Escape from Ambiguity

Despite the efforts of a new generation of popularisers, many sociologists of science have diagnosed that the institution of science is currently in a crisis of trust. One of the reasons for this is the widespread politicisation, economisation and challenge of scientific knowledge by alternative facts. In my view, there are three ways to tackle this problem. The first way is to take an epistemically conservative position and understand scientific facts in a very reductionist way. This path, as I have shown, is taken by individuals like Dawkins or Kutschera. They aim to distinguish "good science" from what, in their eyes, is "bad science". Yet, this leads them to underestimate, and in some cases, even defy both the complexity of the world and the diversity of scientific knowledge production. The second way is to strive for a democratisation of knowledge production. This path is currently being pursued by many scientific institutions. The third way, which I would like to explore in the case studies of this book, is to embrace the diversity of scientific knowledge not only in the form of lip service, or via diversity programmes, but also by recognising that epistemic diversity is an important component of scientific practice and its communication.

The entanglement of science and society can best be depicted as a relational history. From such a perspective, cooperation and participation appear to be the norm, while a sharp delineation of certified experts and laypersons was a special characteristic of the late nineteenth and early twentieth century (Nikolow and Schirrmacher 2007). With responsible science, public science and citizen science, both societal sub-systems, seem to re-enter their former, participatory, *modus operandi*. When modern science was developed between the seventeenth and nineteenth centuries, it was an open and public enterprise. Science spectacles and public experiments of the *ancien régime* prove this. And, even the networking activities of Charles Darwin, Alfred Russel Wallace, Gregor Mendel, and Carl Linnaeus show how public science really was. Hence, all these scientists, who are nowadays celebrated as individual geniuses, depended on broad networks of local providers of information, who were recruited from all social strata. The aim of this kind of science was to unfold the book of nature by gathering as many natural-historical information as possible.

A first demarcation occurred in the second half of the nineteenth century. In this period, many sciences transitioned from a dense description of reality to an experimental practice in which the investigation of causes and effects advanced the ideal of undisturbed test conditions. Individual local descriptions were no longer required, but rather a specified and reproducible knowledge for dealing with highly complex experimental systems. For ordinary citizens, the access to this elaborated world became increasingly difficult. Around 1900, science began implicitly adapting more and more to a reliance on the working concept of division of labour. Much of the technological success (and horrors) in the twentieth century seems to be a result of this division. Gradually, the nimbus of scientists as producers of clear and objective knowledge developed. Specialisation and experimentalisation, however, led to a functional alienation from the public. This alienation, in turn led to the emergence of the image of a distinct "truth cast". The public was now framed as audience and no more as co-producers. Scientists were, among other things, depicted in their media representation as Janus-faced. Science and scientists could be as frightening as Stanley Kubrick's "Dr. Strangelove", but also particularly inviting and trustworthy, as (for example) the German animal expert and popular-scientist Bernhard Grzimek or the French adventurer Jacques Cousteau. Institutional science and its popularisers stood for objective and instructive knowledge but this knowledge was also perceived sometimes as something esoteric, sometimes even frightening.

In the second half of the twentieth century, politicians "discovered" science as a decision-making resource for questions about the implementation of new technologies in society. Scientists have now been framed as experts for topics such as nuclear power, genetic engineering, and so on. The political system expected from the scientific system to produce clear statements to generate a capacity to act in relation to specific technology related issues. However, science gained the same degree of complexity and diversity as it had acquired credibility as source for (at least rhetorically) unambiguous knowledge. In the 1980s and 1990s, this led to a system-related disenchantment of public expectations in science and a shattering of trust in the (western) "truth cast" itself. This disillusionment became evident, for example, in the Europe-wide discussions on the consequences of Chernobyl, but also in the discourse about climate-change beginning in the 1990s. When "suddenly", those from whom clear statements about knowledge were expected fought out public disputes and interpreted the data material available to them in different ways, the public trust in expertise was shaken. In addition a self-confident critique rose in western societies towards the implementation of science related technologies like genetic engineering as well as the communication of their consequences. In general, a linear deficit model of science and society prevailed. Some produce, spread and explain knowledge (scientists), the citizens (whose everyday life in modern societies is determined by this knowledge) are conceptualised as passive recipients. On the basis of scientific knowledge, however, decisions (by politicians) were framed as haven been made in "their interest". The anti-nuclear power movement, science shops and other citizen driven (or as "for" citizens framed) actions were the first initiatives that reacted to this paternalistic conception of dissemination, explanation and decision making. According to the sociologist Peter Weingart, since the turn towards the twenty-first century the institution of science has become aware that the paternalistic implications of its public conception no longer fit into the political culture characterised by democratic claims about participation. The "Public Engagement in Science and Technology" program in the US and the UK and the "Science in Dialogue" program in Germany of the 2000s were the first dialogical (but not yet fully "participatory") reactions to this crisis (Weingart 2001). In times of growing uncertainty, fostered by the financial crisis of 2008, the climate crisis, and the growing social inequality in almost all societies, many people are looking for something stable and secure. What would be better suited for this than science? Yet, as I will show in the following sections of this book a stiff, cold, and overly simplified understanding of scientific knowledge production may not be suited for this task. On the contrary, it can contribute to the emergence of precisely those anti-scientific epistemic strategies that many "pro-science hardliners" are trying to combat.

2.5 Populism and Participation: Two Sides of the Same Coin

In April 2020, at the height of the first wave of the Covid-19 pandemic, something extraordinary occurred in the United States. President Donald Trump's son-in-law and senior adviser Jared Kushner bragged during an interview with the Washington Post's journalist Bob Woodward about how President Trump had taken the country and its crisis response "back from the doctors" (Warren et al. 2020). When Kushner made this statement the government had just published guidelines for the reopening of the states. Against the backdrop of this program, entitled "Opening Up America Again", the president immediately tweeted "LIBERATE MICHIGAN," "LIBERATE MINNESOTA," and "LIBERATE VIRGINIA" in response to experts advising to maintain the stay-at-home orders in those states. For his supporters, the case was clear that both the CDC and other medical institutions would exaggerate the pandemic and use it to consolidate their own oppressive power. Democratic Governor Gretchen Widmer and leading epidemiology expert Dr. Anthony Faucci appeared in this depiction as sinister figures endangering the freedom of the American people. I could have simply overlooked this episode as one of the countless extravagances of Trump administration. Yet, it remained in my consciousness because it underscores one of the most comprehensive socio-political and epistemic transformations of twenty-first century societies.

Macromodels of social theory such as the "information society" (Wiener 1948), the "risk society" (Beck 2003 (=1986)) or the "knowledge society" (Weingart 2001) have disappeared from the focus of science and technology studies in recent years. They have been replaced by studies that examine the development of science and society from a meso- or even micro-perspective (e.g. Latour 2002). Although I regard such small-scale, mosaic-like approaches fruitful and important in our fragmented and highly complex contemporary societies, it also seems important to me to pause from time to time and to combine the many relevant findings and narratives in the vast field of science and technology studies with a broad brushstroke. The concepts I want to utilise in this section of the book are "trust", "knowledge" and "power". Against the background of the interplay of these components, I will draw a picture of our societies that reveals the tendency that both policies and individual action are increasingly based on the assumption that many people have lost confidence in their decision-making and knowledge institutions. I will further show that political and scientific elites, as well as many disenchanted citizens, are seeking a way out of this real or perceived crisis of trust by elevating the concept of "participation" narratively to the status of a saviour. It matters less how participation is conceived and on which levels it is enabled (i.e. who demands it, who profits, or who offers it). For many actors the focus is rather on the performative practice of joint action. For others, it is mere self-interest. In some cases participation even seems to serve as a mere substitute for the partition of power when making decisions.

Widely praised, demanded, implanted, and presumed in institutional contexts (from international science policy agencies to local environmental initiatives) participation in the production of knowledge is oftentimes performed as if it is an end pf itself and not a tool to achieve larger societal objectives. A praised "politically correct precondition," but one that often remains strangely underdetermined in its meaning and direction (Mahr et al. 2018): more a phrase that thrives on the countercultural semblance of the activism of the late 1960s and 1970s than a progressive program that helps democratise knowledge and decisions about its implementation (Mahr 2017). In addition, many participatory programs of this kind are not really inclusive upon closer inspection. Hence, they address a predominantly formally educated, rather affluent section of the population. This is, for example, the case with many digital citizen science projects (Mahr and Dickel 2019; Strasser et al. 2019). This blind spot was not left unfilled. This becomes evident by studying another complementary form of participation, which emerges from the darker corners of the internet, the far-right political spectrum, as well as disenfranchised social groups. The motto of such groups is "to trust only that of which you yourself are a part!". Not only did Donald Trump, his son-in-law, and his other followers ride this wave, but also "epistemically alternative movements" be they progressive, conservative or considered wacky like contemporary flat earth enthusiasts who are very active on social media platforms like Instagram or YouTube.

The figurehead of modern flat earth enthusiasts, Mark Sargent, expressed this attitude at the first Canadian Flat-Earth Conference (Edmonton, Alberta) in 2018 as follows: "For the (…) scientific community I bear a message, I like science… (but) you have taken what should have been simple observations and twisted them to your needs. We are the new scientists" (Brewis 2019). In this light, populism based on mistrust in both scientific and political institutions and public participation might be two sides of the same coin. The central question becomes: how can the fundamental problem that is expressed both in populism and in current participation efforts be resolved?

The amazing thing about the new Flat Earth enthusiasts organising and exchanging themselves on internet platforms like YouTube and Reddit is an admirable seriousness. In contrast to the strange Flat Earth societies of the late nineteenth century and the comedic social media accounts of early Web 2.0, individuals like Sargent take not only the belief in a flat earth seriously but also the scientific method. As the prominent science and media YouTuber hbomberguy in his splendid video "Flat Earth: A Measured Response" states: "These people are progressives. They believe in science, and reason, and evidence. They want to move the understanding of the earth forwards (…)" (Ibid). Two things guide this growing community: the diffuse feeling that the institutions of science and their allies are keeping something from all of us and that science as a practice has alienated itself from its epistemic roots. For Sargent and his companions there can therefore only be one epistemic strategy. The people must take science back into their own hands. As the retired neurosurgeon and 17th United States Secretary of Housing and Urban Development Ben Carson framed it in 2015: "the ark was built by amateurs, the Titanic by experts" (Lee 2015). Might the same be true for a new, a people's cosmology?

Most modern flat earth enthusiasts perceive abstract models, mathematical calculations, or mediated representations of the world as tools of possible deception. To be accepted as truth, such information must be translated, shared and believed (by the recipient's side). But what if the people who generate and disseminate this knowledge have lost my trust?

Testimonial knowledge can only ever be as credible as the person conveying it. Have not the sciences demonstrated over and over again that they disagree and compete among each other, that there are corrupt individuals in their ranks who work with big pharmaceutical companies or the tobacco industry? Haven't scientific advancements such as in "green genetics" (GMO) deprived many ordinary people, honest working farmers for example, of their livelihood or worse yet forced the shackles of patented seeds on them? In a world, where literally everything is beyond your control, cracking the "real" answer, as Jared Bauer in his video review of the Netflix documentary "Behind the curve" (2019) states, "(…) is appealing" (Bauer 2019). Questioning together with others a given but as opaque perceived truth might create the feeling that the world is (in a nostalgic way) rational and predictable.

To this end, modern flat earthers are reviving the idea of *direct realism* (or, as some say, naive empiricism). Direct realism is the idea that directly (via the own senses) perceived objects are external objects, qualities, facts, or events. In other words; the world is basically as we perceive it (see Fig. 2.1). Therefore, no translation is needed, no outside experts with their presumed agendas need to be trusted. However weak the evidence produced by the Flat Earth community may appear from the outside, it is both *empirical* and *communal* and therefore perceived as valid from within the community. This applies, to their easily replicable (and as well to debunk) measurements of the curvature of the earth, the study of flight patterns of passenger aircrafts or their repetitive form of communication on social media. Against this backdrop, flat earth science may appear to some individuals as a superior epistemic and social strategy, as it operationalises the myth of epistemic neutrality propagated by old fashioned science.

The communal nature of Flat Earth activities is central to understanding the movement. Participation and joint activity to uncover a hidden or concealed truth is at the centre. One's epistemic activities are directed against the supposedly powerful and one's own participation is understood as a protest. In this, the modern Flat Earth enthusiasts also resemble other modern anti-establishment movements with epistemic pretensions such as the anti-vaccinationists or even the infamous QAnon conspiracy. In her excellent lead story in the June issue of The Atlantic,

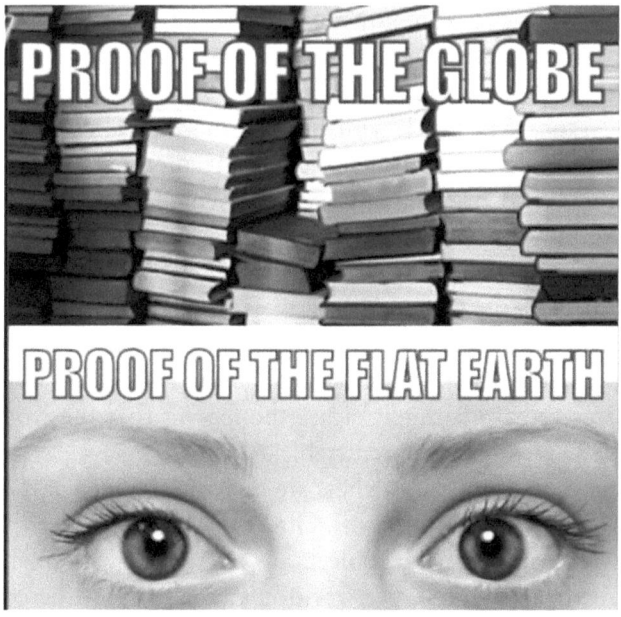

Fig. 2.1 Flat Earth Meme: https://www.reddit.com/r/facepalm/comments/gfqhtn/a_flat_earther_made_this_surprisingly_accurate/ (visited: 12. December 2020)

Executive Editor Adrienne LaFrance describes QAnon as a "real-time participatory conspiracy theory" (LaFrance 2020). For her, QAnon is "emblematic of modern America's susceptibility to conspiracy theories" (Ibid), like those centring around Area 51, the assassination of JFK or "Pizza Gate". She adds that the movement would have grown beyond "a loose collection of conspiracy-minded chat room inhabitants" and inspired real world actions that resemble cult like behaviour (Ibid). As a science and technology studies scholar with an interest in social movements, I could not agree more. However, LaFrance also characterises QAnon as a "movement united in mass rejection of reason, objectivity, and other enlightenment values" (Ibid). In this respect, however, I disagree with her. As in the case of modern Flat Earth enthusiasts, the truth seems to me to be more complex. In my opinion, QAnon also operates in the mode of naïve empiricism. The supporters of the Q-movement consider themselves to be exposers of hidden truths: truths, concealed by the political, economic and scientific elites. Their participatory practice centres around the analysis of so-called "Q-Drops". Such "drops" are framed by the Q-community as encrypted messages left for them on 4Chan to decipher by an individual (Q) who claims to be an insider of the so called "deep state" and its sinister doings. If we look at the collaborative analysis of these messages from the angle of an epistemic strategy, it becomes clear that "truth", "experience", and "community" are understood as guiding principles of QAnon. For example, followers of Q are focused on collectively exposing the supposed truth about Covid19, making sense of the policy decisions of political actors (for example, state wide lockdowns) or the recommendations of academic elites like Dr. Anthony Faucci. Both are seen by the followers of Q as distant from the empirical everyday experience of many Americans: the economic reality of a life from pay check to pay check or the experienced disenfranchisement of those living in rural regions. In this context, the analysis of Q can be understood as a collaborative search for meaning and truth utilising methods that resemble scientific or forensic puzzle solving. It represents the desire to reduce the complexity of a world that is seen as too confusing and over which the individual can have little influence. It is about (re)gaining a feeling of control and knowledge.

An analogous situation exists with the numerous conspiracy theories surrounding the SARS-CoV-2 pandemic and the distribution of the first COVID19 vaccines since December 2020. A widely distributed "viral" video by a European-based group called World Doctors Alliance combines, for example, voices of self-proclaimed experts (predominantly family doctors) who cast doubt on the existence of SARS-CoV-2, the effectiveness and the safety of COVID19 vaccines with an appeal to all "ordinary and liberty loving people of the world" to do "their own sceptical research" (see Dupuy and Joffe-Block 2020). The "experts" appearing in the video have neither an epidemiological nor a virological background. Rather, they make their individual experience known and mix the real risks of an active substance developed in record time with the idea of a pharmaceutical world conspiracy. Their oft-repeated call for viewers to do their own research focuses more on generating an "us versus the elites" feeling than on what methods might actually be available to the general population to do immunological research at home. Research in this sense may be limited to googling videos and participating in forum discussions.

Given this reality, participation and populism tend to overlap. Political approaches that strive to appeal to ordinary people who feel that their concerns are unheard and disregarded by established elites tend to create outside and inside groups. On the one side of the aisle, they allege, is the "swamp" of political elites and their servants in science and economy, while on their side are the honest ordinary people, who are seeking simple truths and unity. This unity and truth must be achieved by a process of collaboration, of uncovering of secrets and by refuting forms of knowledge that are against the interest of a discursively created "us". To "make America great again" means therefore also to produce a new kind of accessible knowledge, from the people and by the people. The epistemic strategies of the Flat Earth enthusiasts, the QAnon conspiracy, or anti-vaccinationists also have an aesthetic function. As in the case of classical epistemology advocated by philosophers Karl Popper and Thomas Kuhn, these new social-epistemic movements emphasise ideas such as cognitive simplicity and productive virtue. Just as modern art is devalued as cranky or scatological and contrasted with the idealistic realism of a Thomas Kinkade or Jon McNaughton, so too are simple explanations that mimic the naïve ideal of the scientific method. They are favoured in such movements over the perceived abstract and inaccessible approaches of institutional science.

However, the demand to participate in the production of scientific knowledge by social groups who feel disenfranchised does not always align with populist politics. This is the case, for example, in the epistemic activities of the women's health movement, the civil rights movement, the HIV movement or popular approaches towards epidemiology. Unlike the Flat Earth enthusiasts or the QAnon conspiracy theorists, these groups do not rally behind the idea that a vague elite is withholding basic truths from them. Rather, they gather concrete evidence that their (bodily) experiences are not represented in the scientific or medical system. As the sociologists Michel Callon and Vololona Rabeharisoa point out, such movements emerge under specific socio-epistemic conditions and aim to "impose a new form of articulation between scientific research and political identities", thereby "linking the issues of research content and results to that of their place in (…) (society)" (Callon and Rabeharisoa 2007). Therefore, these groups are more concerned with participation and representation than with positioning themselves as a counter-model to the institutional sciences. In the next chapter, I will take a closer look at the role of experiential knowledge for the project of a more inclusive and diverse science.

2.6   Experiential Knowledge: A New Chance for Epistemic Diversity?

Since the late nineteenth century, the professionalisation of science and medicine as well as the growing dominance of the experimental sciences have created a growing divide between professionals producing scientific and medical knowledge in specialised institutions and a lay public. The lay public is often characterised as consuming the products of science and medicine. The authority of science and medicine did not go uncontested, but overall, the authoritative knowledge became increasingly associated with the scientific gaze and a set of epistemic norms, including objectivity, precision, and quantification (Strasser and Mahr 2017). Such norms expressed the hardening of the distinction between experience and experiment which had previously been so important in the making of modern science and the growing exclusion of experience as a legitimate source of scientific knowledge. Although experiential knowledge was still essential for experimental virtuosity, it was made invisible when the results of such experiments were published. In some fields, especially in natural history, it was still possible well into the twentieth century to claim that experiential knowledge and personal subjectivity were legitimate sources of scientific knowledge. However, they increasingly became rather rare epistemic strategies (Strasser et al. 2019).

In current participatory research, conducted within the scope of scientific institutions (e.g. digital citizen science), the challenges to the monopoly of expert knowledge, both experimental and clinical, rests in part on the claim that lay people's experience of their own bodies and environments can be reliable sources of scientific knowledge (Mahr and Dickel 2019). The ability of lay people to identify changes in their bodies, as citizen scientists for example, rests on intimate bodily experiences. Their epistemic groundings is founded in the intimacy of bodily perceptions. It is not reason at work, but knowing one's own body; not objective facts, but subjective sensations; not cold experiments, but individual experience. A prominent example for the rising trust in experiential knowledge is the "lithium study" lead by the ALS (amyotrophic lateral sclerosis) community, which is part of the online social health network PatientsLikeMe (PLM). As in the year 2008 an Italian research group published a paper that claimed that the oral or intravenous intake of Lithium delays the progression of ALS symptoms (Fornai et al. 2008). Patients from all over the world were enthusiastic and hopeful about the promised possibility to slow down the development of their progressive nerve disease.

Yet, from within the only community of PLM discussion and doubt emerged towards the study of Fornai and his colleagues. Not only was the sample size (16 treated patients in a single blind trial) discussed but also the claim itself, hence, the experiences of the 348 ALS patients registered at PLM during this time seemed to contradict it. Most of them were already using nutritional supplements, including lithium, and felt no significant difference in their illness experience. Therefore, a small group of them had the idea to do their own experience-based study. For this they developed an online spreadsheet to gather more reliable data about the effect of lithium, circulated it, and asked the other PLM patients within the network to take part in a patient driven study. For this the community members began to take the drug off-label via their family doctors and reported their experiences with lithium regularly. With this methodology of self-observation and self-reporting the community (which was later supported by digital tools of PLM itself) found 12 months after beginning the treatment no effect of lithium on the progression of ALS (Wicks et al. 2011). In this example, experiential knowledge of patients served as a corrective for a small single blind trial lead by professional scientists (Mahr 2017).

Although experiential knowledge has been most directly been associated with sensations of one's own body, it can also refer to knowledge that foregrounds bodily sensations of the outer world, rather than measurements performed by instruments for example. When lay people provide supporting evidence for a protein structure on the popular participatory science platform FoldIt, they frequently refer to their "feeling" for the correct structure and their "experience" with the protein. This is what an editorialist for Nature called "science by intuition". How can such epistemic strategies be considered legitimate science, knowing that the very exclusion of experiential knowledge was part of the making of modern science? Yet, such ways of producing scientific knowledge did not arise spontaneously within participatory online research projects, but followed directly from the challenges to the authority of science by lay people, not scientists, in the 1960 and 1970s (Strasser and Mahr 2017). In the turmoil of the counterculture, activists challenging the authority of science attempted to reclaim bodily experience as a legitimate source of scientific knowledge, in order to relocate the distribution of power and knowledge, reopening the epistemological toolbox of science along the way.

Such strategies at the intersection of social activism, health, science and politics are currently experiencing a renaissance. Their resurrection indicates that the crisis of confidence of significant societal groups towards political and scientific institutions is not only leading to a narrowing or simplification of epistemic strategies, as the conservatism of many popular scientists and conspiracy theorists alike might suggest. Rather, the rise of experiential knowledge can also be understood as a participatory corrective to institutional medicine and science. A corrective that, if wisely incorporated, could help bring science closer to its own ideal of multiperspectivity. This experiential diversity is not exhausted in mere tokenism but is also able to reform the core of scientific knowledge production: the sphere of epistemic values. Both classical and modern complementary epistemic social movements can be understood, from an empirical perspective, as practical attempts to implement new scientific values. The work of the feminist philosopher Helen Longino in particular points in this direction (Longino 1990, 1997). Longino complements the classical scientific values analysed by Thomas Kuhn (accuracy, consistency, scope, simplicity and fruitfullness) with diversity values. Such epistemological values are: empirical adequacy, novelty, ontological heterogeneity, complexity of interaction, applicability to human needs and diffusion of power (Willmes 2013). If we understand diversity as a conscious and reflexive approach to the diversity of forms of knowledge in society, then it can become an organisational as well as socio-political concept for a different kind of science. A science that propagates an appreciative, conscious, and respectful handling of diversity and individuality of people, their experiences, and their attempts to solve problems. Diversity as an epistemic tool is not oriented towards deficits but towards the experiences of people which can be made comprehensible and usable as potential for human knowledge. In this context, it is also important to re-situate the role of facts, both in their classical epistemic form (as secure knowledge), as discursive quantities that can become politically or culturally powerful, or as social things that stabilise and configure social realities.

Such an understanding of epistemic diversity might help us to understand our own understanding of knowledge in a more systematic and context sensitive way. In certain settings diversity might refer to the idea that the production of scientific knowledge depends on social positions. Therefore, an appropriate strategy would be to include researchers from diverse social backgrounds, genders, racial and ethnic backgrounds into science. Yet, in other settings it might become more important to emphasise and foster different styles of reasoning to advance the production of scientific knowledge. Such modes of diversity in knowledge production interact with lived experience and provide it with an epistemically relevant frame of reference. The following three case studies (Chaps. 3, 4 and 5) explore this interconnectedness in greater detail, revealing a new horizon for socially relevant epistemic activity that reconfigure both our understanding of expertise and the production of factual knowledge.

References

Alvarez-Salvado, Efren, Vincente Pallares, Andrea Moreno, and Santiago Canals. 2014. Functional MRI of Long-Term Potentiation: Imaging Network Plasticity. *Philosophical Transactions of the Royal Society B* 369 (1633). https://doi.org/10.1098/rstb.2013.0152.

Bauer, Jared (Wisecrack). 2019. *Flat Earth: What Makes REAL Science - Wiserack Edition. Youtube Video Essay.* https://www.youtube.com/watch?v=umo6pMCkcXs. Accessed 25 July 2021.

Beck, Ulrich. 2003 (=1986). *Risikogesellschaft.* Frankfurt a. M.: Suhrkamp.

Boyle, Peter, Nigel Gray, Jack Henningfield, John Seffrin, and Witold A. Zatonski, eds. 2010. *Tobacco. Science, Policy, and Public Health.* 2nd ed. Oxford: Oxford University Press.

Brewis, Harry (@hbomberguy). 2019. Flat Earth: A Measured Response. *YouTube.*www.youtube.com/watch?v=2gFsOoKAHZg. Accessed 9 Dec 2020.

Callon, Michel, and Rabeharisoa Vololona. 2007. The Growing Engagement of Emergent Concerned Groups in Political and Economic Life: Lessons from the French Association of Neuromuscular Disease Patients. *Science, Technology, & Human Values* 33 (2): 230–261.

Carpenter, Morgan. 2018. Intersex Variations, Human Rights, and the International Classification of Diseases. *Health and Human Rights* 20 (2): 205–214.

ChoGlueck, Christopher. 2017. *What Are Scientific Facts? SciU Conversations in Science at Indiana University.* https://blogs.iu.edu/sciu/2017/10/31/what-are-scientific-facts/. Accessed 9 Dec 2020.

Daston, Lorraine. 2001. Objektivität und die Flucht aus der Perspektive. In *Wunder, Beweise und Tatsachen. Zur Geschichte der Rationalität,* ed. Lorraine Daston, 127–156. Frankfurt a. M.: Fischer.

Daston, Lorraine, and Peter Galison. 2010. *Objectivity.* Cambridge: Zone Books.

Dawkins, Richard. 2015. Is It a Theory? *Is It a Law? No, It's A Fact.*https://www.richarddawkins.net/2015/11/is-it-a-theory-is-it-a-law-no-its-a-fact/. Accessed 9 Dec 2020.

Dupuy, Beatrice, and Jude Joffe-Block. 2020. Video Contains a Litany of False Claims About COVID-19 and Vaccines. *AP News*, December 10.https://apnews.com/article/fact-checking-afs:Content:9837440018. Accessed 9 Dec 2020.

Ehrlich, Paul, and Rudolph Gonder. 1914. *Experimentelle Chemotherapie.*https://www.pei.de/SharedDocs/Downloads/DE/institut/veroeffentlichungen-von-paul-ehrlich/1906-1914/1914-experimentelle-chemotherapie.pdf?__blob=publicationFile&v=2. Accessed 9 Dec 2020.

Fausto-Sterling, Anne. 1993. The Five Sexes: Why Male and Female Are Not Enough. *The Sciences* 33 (2).: 20p.

———. 2012. *Sex/Gender. Biology in a Social World.* New York: Routledge.

Fausto-Sterling, Anne, and Edward Stein. 2004 (=2000). *Sexing the Body: Gender Politics and the Construction of Sexuality.* New York: Basic Books.

Fleck, Ludwik. 2017 (=1935). *Entstehung und Entwicklung einer wissenschaftlichen Tatsache,* Frankfurt a. M.: Suhrkamp.

Fornai, Francesco, Patrizia Longone, Luisa Camaro, Olga Kastsichuenka, Michaela Ferrucci, Michaela Laura Manca, Gloria Lazzeri, Alida Spalloni, Nastacia Bellio, Paola Lenzu, Gabriele Modugno, Isodoro Siciliano, Murri Ciro, Stefano Ruggieri, and Antonio Paparelli. 2008. Lithium Delays Progression of Amyotrophic Lateral Sclerosis. *Oric National Academy of Sciences USA* 105 (6): 16404–16407.

IPCC. 2014. *AR5 Climate Change 2014: Impacts, Adaption, and Vulnerability.* https://www.ipcc.ch/report/ar5/wg2/. Accessed 18 Dec 2020.

Kutschera, Ulrich. 2018. *Das Gender-Paradoxon: Mann und Frau als evolvierte Menschentypen.* Münster: LIT Verlag.

LaFrance, Adrienne. 2020. The Prophecies of Q. American Conspiracy Theories Are Entering a Dangerous New Phase. *The Atlantic* (online). https://www.theatlantic.com/magazine/archive/2020/06/qanon-nothing-can-stop-what-is-coming/610567/. Accessed 30 Dec 2020.

Latour, Bruno. 2002. *Die Hoffnung der Pandora: Untersuchungen zur Wirklichkeit der Wissenschaft.* Frankfurt a. M: Suhrkamp.

Lee, Timothy B. 2015. *Ben Carson: The Ark was Built by Amateurs, the Titanic by Professionals.* Vox. https://www.vox.com/policy-and-politics/2015/10/29/9639228/ben-carson-noahs-ark. Accessed 25 July 2021.

Longino, Helen. 1990. *Science as Social Knowledge: Values and Objectivity in Scientific Inquiry.* Princeton: Princeton University Press.

———. 1997. Feminist Epistemology as Local Epistemology. *Proceedings of the Aristotelian Society, Supplementary Volumes* 71: 19–35, & 37–54.

Magubane, Zine. 2014. Spectacles and Scholarship: Caster Semenya, Intersex Studies, and the Problem of Race in Feminist Theory. *Journal of Women in Culture and Society* 39 (3). https://doi.org/10.1086/674301.

Mahr, Dana. 2017. Self-Reporting and Participatory Health Platforms: Empowerment Through Sharing Information About Oneself Online? *Harvard Bill of Health.* https://blog.petrieflom.law.harvard.edu/2017/05/01/self-reporting-and-participatory-health-platforms-empowerment-through-sharing-information-about-oneself-online/. Accessed 18 Dec 2020.

Mahr, Dana, and Livia Prüll. 2018. Körperliche Selbstermächtigung aus dem 3D-Drucker? Feministische Kulturen als Parallelwelten und der Kampf um gesellschaftliche Teilhabe seit 1970. In *Kybernetik, Kapitalismus, Revolutionen. Emanzipatorische Perspektiven im technologischen Wandel,* ed. Paul Buckermann, Anne Koppenburg, and Simon Schaub, 161–190. Münster: Unrast.

Mahr, Dana, and Sascha Dickel. 2019. Citizen Science Beyond Invited Participation: Nineteenth Century Amateur Naturalists, Epistemic

Autonomy, and Big Data Approaches Avant La Lettre. *History and Philosophy of the Life Sciences* 41 (4).

Mahr, Dana, Claudia Göbel, Alan Irwin, and Katrin Vohland. 2018. Watching or Being Watched – Enhancing Productive Discussion Between the Citizen Sciences, the Social Sciences and the Humanities. In *Citizen Science: Innovation in Open Science, Society and Policy*, ed. Susanne Hecker, Muki Haklay, Anne Bowser, Zen Makuch, and Johannes Vogel. London: UCL Press. https://doi.org/10.14324.

Marshall, Eliot. 1987. Tobacco Science Wars; the Industry Has Been Bullying Scientists, According to Researchers Who Lead the Campaign Against Environmental Tobacco Smoke. *Science* 236: 250p.

Nikolow, Sybilla, and Arne Schirrmacher, eds. 2007. *Wissenschaft und Oeffentlichkeit als Ressourcen füreinander. Studien zur Wissenschaftsgeschichte im 20. Jahrhundert*. Frankfurt a. M.: Campus.

Pasquale, Frank. 2015. *The Black Box Society: The Secret Algorithms That Control Money and Information*. Cambridge/London: Harvard University Press.

Rippon, Gina. 2019. *The Gendered Brain. The New Neuroscience that Shatters the Myth of the Female Brain*. London: Vintage Publishing.

Roukos, Dimitrios H. 2012. Longevity with Systems Medicine? Epigenome, Genome and Environment Interactions Network. *Epigenomics* 4 (2): 119–123.

Rubino, Michael. 2015. The Boy with Half a Brain. *Indianapolis Monthly*, December 23. https://www.indianapolismonthly.com/longform/boy-with-half-brain-william-buttars. Accessed 18 Dec 2020.

Shapin, Steven. 2010. *Never Pure. Historical Studies of Science as if It Was Produced by People with Bodies, Situated in Time, Space, Culture, and Society, and Struggling for Credibility and Authority*. Baltimore: Johns Hopkins University Press.

Shapiro, Ben. 2019. *Facts Don't Care About Your Feelings*. Hermosa Beach: Creators Publishing.

Strasser, Bruno J, and Dana Mahr. 2017. Experiential Knowledge, Public Participation, and the Challenge to the Authority of Science in the 1970s. *Harvard Bill of Health*. https://blog.petrieflom.law.harvard.edu/2017/05/02/experiential-knowledge-public-participation-and-the-challenge-to-the-authority-of-science-in-the-1970s/. Accessed 18 Dec 2020.

Strasser, Bruno, Jerome Baudry, Dana Mahr, Gabriela Sanchez, and Elise Tancoigne. 2019. Citizen Science? Rethinking Science and Public Participation. *Science & Technology Studies* 32 (2): 52–76.

Taubert, Marco, Arno Villringer, and Patrick Ragert. 2012. Learning-Related Gray and White Matter Changes in Humans: An Update. *The Neuroscientist* 18 (4): 320–325.

Tavernise, Sabrina. 2017. Ben Shapiro, a Provocative "Gladiator", Battles to Win Young Conservatives. *The New York Times* (online). https://www. nytimes.com/2017/11/23/us/ben-shapiro-conservative.html.   Accessed 18 Dec 2020.

Uebel, Thomas. 2020. Vienna Circle. *Stanford Encyclopedia of Philosophy.* https://plato.stanford.edu/cgi-bin/encyclopedia/archinfo.cgi?entry=vienna-circle. Accessed 18 Dec 2020.

Viloria, Hida, and Maria Nieto. 2020. *The Spectrum of Sex. The Science of Male, Female, and Intersex.* London: Jessica Kingsley Publishers.

von Wahl, Angelika. 2019. From Object to Subject: Intersex Activism and the Rise and Fall of the Gender Binary in Germany, Social Politics. *International Studies in Gender, State & Society.* https://doi.org/10.1093/sp/jxz044. Accessed 18 Dec 2020.

Warren, Michael, Jamie Gangel, and Elizabeth Stuart. 2020. Jared Kushner Bragged in April that Trump Was Taking the Country 'Back from the Doctors'. *CNN Politics.* https://edition.cnn.com/2020/10/28/politics/woodward-kushner-coronavirus-doctors/index.html. Accessed 18 Dec 2020.

Weingart, Peter. 2001. *Die Stunde der Wahrheit. Zum Verhältnis der Wissenschaft zu Politik, Wirtschaft und Medien in der Wissensgesellschaft.* Weilerswist: Velbrück Verlag.

Wicks, Paul, Timothy E. Vaughan, Michael P. Massagli, and James Heywood. 2011. Accelerated Clinical Discovery Using Self-Reported Patient Data Collected Online and a Patient-Matching Algorithm. *Nature Biotechnology* 29 (5): 411–414. Accessed 18 Dec 2020.

Wiener, Norbert. 1948. *Cybernetics: Or Control and Communication in the Animal and the Machine.* Paris: Hermanm & Cie.

Willmes, David. 2013. *Zur Legitimität ethischer und sozialer Werte in der Wissenschaft.* Dissertation Bielefeld. https://pub.uni-bielefeld.de/download/2631123/2631127/Willmes_2013_Zur_Legitimitat_ethischer_und_sozialer_Werte_in_der_Wissenschaft.pdf. Accessed 18 Dec 2020.

World Health Organization, WHO. 2015. *Sexual Health, Human Rights and the Law.* https://apps.who.int/iris/bitstream/handle/10665/175556/9789241564984_eng.pdf;jsessionid=6B51047279C2B0DC7F3B6D1E717DFA58?sequence=1. Accessed 18 Dec 2020.

3

Digital Resilience

Abstract In the context of the digitalisation of disease and health, self-help and health self-care are undergoing a profound transformation. This is particularly evident in the boom in so-called digital health networks, which collect health data from their users in return for providing a community of people with similar conditions. This chapter examines the practice of data "self-reporting" from the perspective of both network providers and people with chronic diseases. A special emphasis is given to the rise of practical resilience of a growing group of users towards the data-centred reduction of their illness experiences.

Keywords Illness experience • Self-reporting • Big-data • Online health platforms • DIY health

During the time of my secondary school years in rural Germany I had a friend. His name was Nico. Nico seemed, in the eyes of us other kids, sometimes strange, introvert and sorrowful. In times of sorrow, his grades in school decreased rapidly. Also, his social behaviour changed sometimes to a degree that made it hard to spend time with him. One day, on such time, my mother informed me that Nico would stay with us for some weeks since his mother, a single parent, needed to have a surgery for her Crohn's disease and he had no other place to go. When I asked my mother about it, she explained that Crohn's is a "disease of the head, that manifests in the bowel". She added that an extraordinary amount of stress is causing it, especially in those who couldn't cope with certain experiences in their lives. During his stay, I talked a lot with Nico to figure out why he seemed so strange from time to time. Soon, he was sharing stories about his mother and all the pain they had been recently going through. Not only was the disease itself giving them a hard time, but also the societal toll of it. The people in our small village were talking about them, he explained with tears in his eyes. Nico recalled the questions: "What kind of mother is this who leaves her son behind in the supermarket only for going to the toilet? What kind of mother misses so many school activities of her kid? What kind of mother would stay inside of her home and isolates herself for weeks just because a little bit of diarrhoea?" A weak person, who doesn't care much, who could be stronger, was their almost consensual verdict. Nico also gave me insight into their daily experiences, and contrary to what the outside view suggested, I got the impression of a mother-son-team of extraordinary strength, facing daily struggles without giving up. I understood that Nico had to fulfil the role of a caregiver in this single parent family; a role that had cost him some success in school and led to both misunderstanding and social isolation in our village given the fact that there was no other person suffering from a similar condition (at least not in the public eye).

Since then, a lot has changed for people living with Crohn's disease, ulcerative colitis, and many other chronic diseases. Much of this has to do with the advancements in the bio-molecular sciences but even more is related to rapid developments in digitalisation of health and illness (see Høivik et al. 2012; Rochelle and Fidler 2012; Kalafateli et al. 2013; Garcia-Sanjuan et al. 2016; Mahr 2017; Mahr et al. 2019; Martinez et al. 2017). If one follows popular narratives, we are even entering new age of both self-help and visibility of chronically ill individuals (Willis and Royne 2017). Gone are the days in which persons like Nico's mother had to suffer in isolation. New participatory online self-help and health platforms like CureTogether, PatientsLikeMe, or Ben's Friends promise their potential subscribers to become part of a support system of communities of people with shared experiences, and the ability to participate actively in the betterment of their condition, while helping scientists find new cures. Yet, this brave new world of community and participation comes with a price. This price is paid in the form of sharing crucial information about one's own health and by (voluntarily or involuntarily) participating in the making of a fundamental shift in how medical knowledge is produced, disseminated, and accessed. Both are not necessarily in the interest of patients and their families, or even society as a whole. They are linked to unique new challenges on an individual, political and epistemological level fostered by commercial actors. The aim of this chapter is therefore to examine to what extent the constantly diversifying culture of online self-help aimed at patients with chronic and (or) rare diseases is transforming our understanding of health and illness. Particular attention will be paid to the infrastructures of such digital (often for-profit) services. The focus will be on both, their interaction with the values and standards of our health care systems and how they (both implicitly and explicitly) contribute to the emergence of alternative social health collectives.

3.1 The Third Wave of Self-Help Culture

Since the late 1960s, health activism and self-help has been a transformative force in how we as a society understand health, illness, care and prevention. Under the banner of self-help, groups that were once marginalised have not only generated visibility in political or medical terms, but have also become actors in the exploration of their own bodies and psyches. In doing so, they provide insights that would not have been possible from the restricted perspective of the medical-scientific system of their time. The achievements of the early Women's Health Movement and ActUP activists during the HIV-AIDS crisis of the 1980s are exemplarily for this. Self-organised cervical examinations, menstrual cycle studies outstanding in accuracy and documentation as well as the critical first-hand influence on drug studies mark this first iteration of transformative self-help culture (Hoffman 1982; Morgen 2002; Epstein 1995; Mahr and Prüll

2018). Socio-formative and epistemological values were physical autonomy and self-determination, the dissolution of knowledge-based power structures in the medical system and (linked to this) the possibility to participate in the generation of new medical and scientific knowledge (FFWHC 1991). At a time when cis-gender white and heterosexual men represented the "human norm" for medical science and "minorities" such as women, queer people, and non-white persons did not find representation in clinical trials, such demands were revolutionary (Frankfort 1973; Nelson 2011). As part of the countercultural movement of the 1960s to 1980s, however, this activism was at the same time in itself biased, being essentially formed by members of the progressive white American middle class. This middle class failed to include intersectional contexts of limited access to health in its activism, which was particularly disadvantageous for black women and queer people of colour among others (e.g. trans* people, intersex people, and sex-workers) from urban centres (Chateuvert 2013). This blindspot still weighs on many countercultural forms of health-related activism and policy approaches even today (Moran 2018).

The second wave of self-help culture, which spanned the 1990s and 2000s, was characterised by a re-integration of self-help movements into the medico-scientific power structures of the health-care system. This process has been described, among others, by the gender studies researcher Tasha N. Dubriwny. In her 2013 book "The Vulnerable Empowered Women. Feminism, Postfeminism and Women's Health" she explored for example the "Go Red for Women" campaign of the American Heart Association of 2009. She shows that such governmental sponsored campaigns adapt the activist language of the Women's Health Movement of the 1970s by evoking themes like empowerment, agency and sisterhood but doesn't share its critical impetus towards institutional knowledge, societal norms, and the healthcare industry. She writes: "Most prominently, unlike (…) the women's health movement, the Go Red campaign prompts a near-unquestioning embracing of medical knowledge and technology. Women's questions about heart disease are answered by medical experts, visually represented on the website as white middle-aged men. The promise of collective action is contradicted by an overall focus on the individual women's responsibility to take care of her own health" (Ibid: 2).

The third wave of self-help culture began in the wake of the financial crisis of 2009 and lasts until to date (see Banner 2017). As the health economy scholars David Stuckler and Sanjay Basu point out (2013), it evolves around the neoliberal (and austerity driven) re-interpretation of self-help as an individual's obligation in relationship to concerned social groups and society in large. Furthermore, its shift to virtual space and the utilisation of Web 2.0 infrastructures is equally characteristic of this trend (Conrad and Stults 2010). In this context, new configurations are emerging between economic interests, national health systems, patients, users, and scientific actors. In the centre of this development are actors like PatientsLikeMe, which I refer to as participatory online health platforms in this paper. Many of these platforms continue, as I will show in the third section, the trend of misusing the language of classical health activism, but combine it with a critique of national health policies and regulatory systems that are presented to potential subscribers as bureaucratic giants that hinder rather than promote medical progress (and thus the health of individuals). An alliance of international companies that operate online health platforms with patients, their families and scientific institutions is implicitly positioned as an alternative to the classic nation-state model. The rationale behind this is that, in exchange for providing a community of like-minded people, users agree to a participatory, targeted collection, donation, storage and the processing of personal health information. During a second step, such information is passed on to third parties often in return for financial compensation (Strasser et al. 2019). As a result, self-help becomes, in part, associated with a hyper-capitalist model of health and research (Mahr 2017).

Much has already been written about what patients and their families actually do on and expect from such platforms including how their experience with such communities impacts both their health behaviour and understanding of illness (e.g. Neal et al. 2006; Grosberg et al. 2016; Magnezi et al. 2014; Lupton 2014). In contrast, research into the profit that such platforms gain from the activities of their subscribers is scarce (Casilli and Gutierrez 2019). Most of the emerging research in this field of study centres around either individual data security or the cultivation of information on such platforms (Janssens et al. 2012; Tempini 2014; Prainsack and Buyx 2017). An overarching perspective that links the connected changes in individual disease identities with the influence of such platforms on health policy, and medical epistemology is still a requisite. The same applies to the resistance of some users/patients towards this trend of commercialisation of self-help. This resistance is expressed in the emergence of new, inclusive and performative local health collectives such as the Spanish GynePunks or open source health networks (Mahr and Prüll 2018).

3.2 Exploring Participatory Online Health Platforms

During the last decade, online health platforms have been rapidly diversified, as Peter Conrad and Cheryl Stults already predicted back in 2010 (Conrad and Stults 2010). Classic health information websites established in the late 1990s and early 2000s, such as WebMD, Mayo Clinic, Healthline, Drugs.com, and Medline Plus focused primarily on providing curated information to those who search online for guidance for health related issues. Commercial portals like WebMD have been harshly criticised, by some, for providing obscure or biased advice, such as the promotion of drugs sold by commercial partners or fostering hypochondria among its users by using alarmist language (Heffernan 2011). As soon as such platforms opened themselves to the users by providing peer-moderated forums (like the 55 sub-communities of WebMD) that foster exchange among information seekers, others began to question the credibility of peer-information that was, produced, discussed, and provided on such platforms (Huh et al. 2016).

Sharing Culture

Nevertheless, this first wave of online health platforms has also paved the way for fundamental changes in today's healthcare culture. They did so by providing non-geographically restricted safe spaces for self-help, advocacy and corporate interests; aspects that seem to contradict themselves but which actually gets bridged in practice. Notably, individuals and populations that are either suffering from very rare conditions such as amyotrophic lateral sclerosis (ALS, as mentioned in Chap. 2) or are living with a disease which is in some cases still societally connected to moral deviancy (e.g. HIV in some parts of Asia) or individual shame (such as inflammatory bowel diseases (IBD)) profit from those virtual spaces. It is not surprising that during the rise of the web 2.0, a new type of online health community was developed oftentimes inspired by and aiming towards the experiences of individuals suffering from rare diseases. The self-proclaimed "non-profit patient network and real time research platform" PatientsLikeMe for example (PatientsLikeMe 2020), narratively links its origins with the life experiences of its co-founder Stephen Heywood, who was diagnosed with ALS in 1998. PatientsLikeMe opened its servers in October 2005 and has, since then, attracted over 600,000 users. Among them are 5862 individuals suffering from Crohn's disease and 2876 persons with ulcerative colitis who share their profiles publicly, including uploaded health information and narratives about their illness experiences. In addition to providing a virtual space in which individuals can discuss their conditions, share their experiences, and connect over related topics, collecting, processing and providing large sets of health information (both for scientific and commercial reasons) has become the main characteristic of the second wave of online health platforms (Mahr 2017). Popular online health networks such as PatientsLikeMe, CureTogether, HealthUnlocked or TrackMyStack use both the language of advocacy and the ethos of online sharing culture to nudge their users into providing all kinds of health related information about themselves. The information oftentimes includes for example SNPs from genetic tests, hospital reports, data from smart devices & fitness trackers as well as in-network generated information (both in form of narratives and survey data) (Ibid). Not too long ago, a call to report this type of information about oneself would have provoked a public outcry by data protectors and possibly actions by policy makers due to the nature of such sensitive info. But with the big data epistemology of personalised or precision medicine on the rise in a globalised world, it seems that the tides have turned. Most platforms are hybrids between commercial enterprises, citizen science projects, social networks, and data-providers for both scientific institutions, governmental actors, and industry established regulatory tools fail to encompass their doings. These tools have been developed to monitor and steer the data usage of institutions that are fully embedded into the medico-scientific system and are therefore, insufficient to cope with the hybrid character of such new platforms. Furthermore, most national regulatory agencies, for example the Federal Office of Public Health in Switzerland, are unable to oversee the activities of social health networks since many health platforms are operating from abroad (see Mahr et al. 2019).

Against the backdrop of sharing culture as a new and idealised form of sociality (see Katrini 2018), PatientsLikeMe and other social health platforms frame the request for the donation of information about one's own health status as a collective responsibility. For them, the accumulation of health data serves a greater good and everybody who shares their own data therefore participates in accomplishing this goal. In April 2016, the PatientsLikeMe blog published under the tag of "Openness Philosophy" the following statement:

> Most healthcare websites have a Privacy Policy. Naturally, we do too. But at PatientsLikeMe, we're more excited about our Openness philosophy. It may sound counterintuitive, but it's what drives our groundbreaking concept. You see, we believe sharing your healthcare experiences and outcomes is good. Why? Because when patients share real-world data, collaboration on a global scale becomes possible. New treatments become possible. Most importantly, change becomes possible. At PatientsLikeMe, we are passionate about bringing people together for a greater purpose: speeding up the pace of research and fixing a broken healthcare system. Currently, most healthcare data is inaccessible due to privacy regulations or proprietary tactics. As a result, research is slowed, and the development of breakthrough treatments takes decades. Patients also can't get the information they need to make important treatment decisions. But it doesn't have to be that way. When you and thousands like you share your data, you open up the healthcare system. You learn what's working for others. You improve your dialogue with your doctors. Best of all, you help bring better treatments to market in record time. PatientsLikeMe enables you to effect a sea change in the healthcare system. We believe that the Internet can democratise patient data and accelerate research like never before. Furthermore, we believe data belongs to you the patient to share with other patients, caregivers,

physicians, researchers, pharmaceutical and medical device companies, and anyone else that can help make patients' lives better. Will you add to our collective knowledge ... and help change the course of healthcare? (Patientslikeme blog 2016)

The promise of collaboratively "fixing a broken healthcare system" and "speeding up the pace of research" seems to be appealing to many who suffer from rare and often misunderstood, stigmatised and/or chronic diseases. The same applies for the various community functions that social health networks are providing. Since 2014 members of the Crohn's community within PatientsLikeMe are, for example, discussing the microbiomic component of their condition. They coordinate among themselves self-experimentation with different diets and even DIY-faecal transplants (see Mahr 2017). Another case of community-based research in social health network involves members of the ALS population on PatientsLikeMe. These highly engaged individuals conducted their own study to fact-check, using their own bodies as experimental agents, the outcomes of a small Italian study, which claimed that aluminium could have a positive effect in slowing down the progress of ALS (Wicks et al. 2011). As it turned out, there was no significant effect of aluminium with respect to the development of the condition (Ibid). Since then, the ALS-study has been used by actors like Paul Wicks, vice president for innovation at PatientsLikeMe, as a showcase for the legitimacy and goodness of the networks activities. He does so even though the communities organised within the network and the practice of data-collection are, if at all, only loosely linked by the community ethos.

The Epistemology of Self-Reporting

To be part of a social health network means to be generous with one's own health information. This seems to be a state of mind which has become deeply embedded into the daily routine of many users of such platforms. The practice of "self-reporting" health related information on online health websites (Strasser et al. 2019) is not only a way for individuals to feel as if they are contributing to the advancement of healthcare, but also a means to be part of a larger community that shares similar bodily and mental experiences. It is not only a tool for corporate interests but has also become a powerful socio-scientific episteme. Only loosely connected to the usage of the French philosopher Michael Foucault (Foucault and Gordon 1980), I understand epistemes here and in the following parts of my article as apparatuses that separate and give value to both statements and practices within a community that is (partly) united by an epistemic *and* social goal. An example would be the advancement of biomedicine and its translation into care. The attraction of "self-reporting" as such an episteme within the online sharing culture is the inescapability of its implied morality. Sharing data is seen as advantageous while withholding is selfish. To partake in the advancement of science and medicine is a social imperative, while anything else is framed as going against the best interests of society. To be part of a health community, therefore contributes to one's own and others mental and physical wellbeing, but it comes at the "low" price of data-donation. A moral economy like this is designed to evoke feelings in possible users such as responsibility (it is my duty to share health information), shame (if I don't share my information others may suffer), or agency (because I share my health information within an online health network I am participating in bettering my own and others situation in the future).

The focus on quantitative (or quantifiable) health information is a telling characteristic of many online patient platforms. The act of sharing intimate bodily information about oneself on commercial platforms might serve scientific, economical, or even political interests. But why do they need to be (mostly) in quantified form? According to the historian of science Theodore M. Porter, the reason for this is connected to some intrinsic and (in the broadest sense) psychological qualities of numbers: We are conditioned to trust them nearly unconditionally. Quantification is a technology of distance and cultural construction of objectivity (Porter 1995). The reliance on numbers and quantitative information minimises disrupting factors such as the need for intimate knowledge and personal trust. Likewise, they are a medium to ensure communication beyond local or cultural boundaries. Numbers reduce complexity into a set of predetermined categories and therefore help to construct a simplified reality of our bodies, identities, social or economic status. Thereby they help others to make supposedly objective decisions about us as individuals or even the course of whole societies (O'Neil 2016; Stuckler and Basu 2013). A decision made with the help of quantified information has the appearance of fairness, impersonality, and egalitarianism. Thus, ultimately enabling the possibility of objective action. Such an epistemic economy of (seemingly) objective data dissolves the individual into the collectivity of large data sets. However, entering my patient data into the database of online health networks not only collectivises me, but also measures and compares my data copy with the information shared by countless others. Ultimately, a data image emerges that has been classified and categorised and can be ported into countless other contexts. Thus, it is not too far-fetched to believe that my daily input of blood pressure values on such a website can eventually have an impact on my credit score, my dating profile, or even my chances of getting a job at a university (Weinberger 2012; Mahr 2017). Of course, the epistemology of self-reporting health data could also contribute to real advances in medical research or individual health as many providers promise. Consequently, we have a double-edged sword to wield when we use such services in private sector but also increasingly in public health-care contexts (Prainsack 2020).

Furthermore it is noteworthy, that the practice of self-reporting encompasses not only data, that has already been quantified by sources outside of these networks (such as SNPs or blood test results), but also includes prospectively quantifiable information co-produced and (statistically) utilised by the providers and their clients. Examples for this are both the DailyMe function of PatientsLikeMe, which asks users to rate their feelings on a daily basis (see Fig. 3.1). Their experience based illness narratives are shared in the network's forums. Although it is still unclear if providers like CureTogether or PatientsLikeMe have already developed the technology necessary to utilise such narratives for their benefits, the rapid development of machine learning algorithms will make it possible in the near future (Yom-Tov 2016).

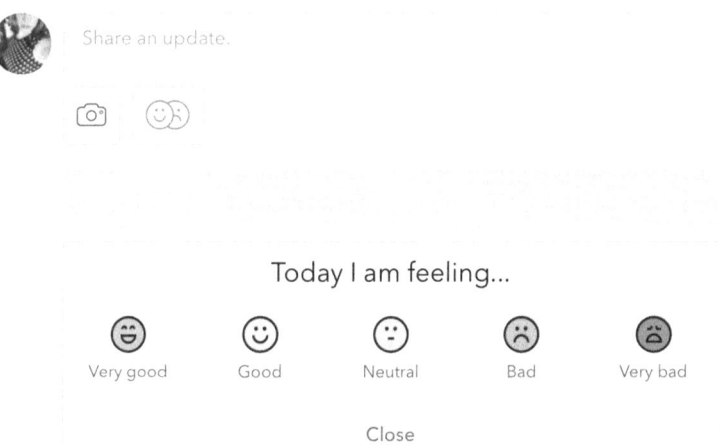

Today I am feeling...

Very good   Good   Neutral   Bad   Very bad

Close

Fig. 3.1   Screenshot of the authors profile page on PatientsLikeMe, Jan 2020

Alternative Platforms

Both commercial and semi-commercial social health networks are currently being challenged. Although many casual users are choosing to become members of the few large commercial or semi-commercial social health networks and community platforms of direct-to-consumer *omics-testing companies, such as uBiome or 23andMe, a wide variety of non-profit and community organised alternatives is emerging. These range from specialised spaces in social aggregation and discussion platforms like Reddit, to highly elaborated data-sharing websites like OpenSNP. In January 2020, the subreddit community r/CrohnsDisease had over 24,500 members discussing and sharing a wide variety of topics, including the *omics of IBD. Some users are even co-analysing each other's phenotypes. That is to say, the observable characteristics of an individual resulting from the interaction between its environment and genotype. This is oftentimes done against the backdrop of detailed knowledge about genomics (r/CrohnsDisease 2020). In the same period of time, OpenSNP attracted about 8000 users and they provided the platform with about 5400 genetic datasets (Greshake-Tzovaras 2020). Among those users, 4771 haven't shared any data yet, while 2904 contributed one phenotype,

1468 users up to ten, 865 more than 20, 329 more than 50 and 123 individuals shared more than 100 datasets (see Fig. 3.2).

According to the co-founders of OpenSNP, the goal of the project is similar to those of both social health networks and direct-to-consumer *omics testing companies, since they also want to provide a platform that helps individuals to understand their own genome better, while at the same time sharing the collected and curated information with the research community for an open and participatory advancement of science. Nevertheless, they reject the idea of monetising this data. In their own words:

> The idea for this project came to Bastian after he was genotyped by 23andMe in May 2011 and started playing around with his data. During his research he became frustrated, because it was not that easy to find more data. He started working on openSNP to fix this. To be clear: This project is not about making money, selling data or to quote Google: "We don't

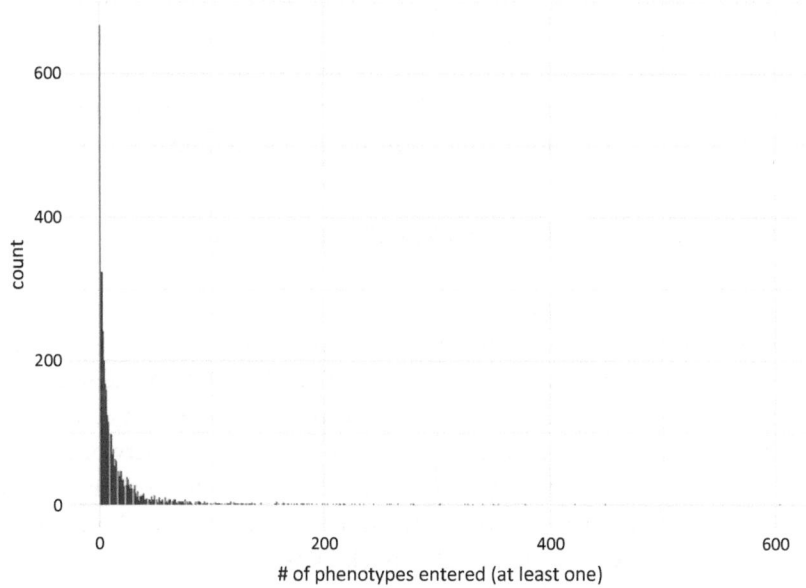

Fig. 3.2 Greshake-Tzovaras (2020)

wanna be evil". We are just interested in making science more open and accessible. (OpenSNP 2020)

OpenSNP and some of its non-profit and commercial competitioners (e.g. Xcode Life, Promethease, Genetic Genie, DNA Land, and Codegene) aim to provide their users with additional and complementary information to the oftentimes limited information and genomic interpretation direct-to-consumer companies are giving to their customers alongside their raw data. The reports or tools for annotation and comparison (e.g. SNPedia) provided by such platforms may for example include gene-nutrition, allergy-susceptibility, or the carrier status for certain genetic conditions. Furthermore, they enable their users to compare their own genomic data and phenotypic expressions with those of other individuals within the site's community. This feature is not common in most community spaces provided by commercial direct-to-consumer genomic testing providers. By taking the ethos of "commons-based peer-production" (the promotion of a non-profit sharing society (see Benkler 2006)) seriously, the founders of OpenSNP prove themselves as tech-savvy digital natives. I suspect therefore, that such platforms are not only created by, but also, utilised by tech-enthusiasts in an disproportionately manner. This usage hints on a digital divide between those who use the more commercial social health networks and those who are searching for alternatives.

Activism in Participatory Online Health Platforms

According to Crohn's and Colitis UK over 5 million people worldwide are experiencing isolation, fear, and embarrassment because of their IBDs (Crohn's and Colitis UK 2015). Many of them also try to make sense out of the aetiology and genetics of their condition (see Wilburn et al. 2017 and Mahr et al. 2019). To become part of an online health network might be a possible way in dealing with both the negative feelings associated with IBD and the patient's quest for understanding, since both might enhance an individual's agency (Prainsack 2014).

But what can agency for someone who suffers from Crohn's disease or ulcerative colitis mean in an online environment? Commonly, social scientists understand agency as an individual's capacity to act independently and to make free choices. As demonstrated in sociological studies, IBDs might have very negative effects on an individual's agency (Wilhelm et al. 2015). During inflammatory periods, individuals with IBD might frequently experience an erosion of their social contacts because they tend to become unable to leave their homes for an extended period of time. Even small tasks like preparing a meal for their family might prove to be an unsolvable task (Mahr et al. 2019). While aware of the chronic nature of their condition, many IBD patients seek to understand their own bodies through the lens of individual illness experiences and provided medical knowledge (Ibid). For an individual that seeks to become actionable towards her/his/their condition, both forms of knowledge tend to be equally valid and important since they are entangled. Medial facts about IBD only make sense when reflected through the lens of one's own individual environmental, nutritional, social, or psychological triggers and first-hand knowledge about the development and time of an episode of IBD. Against this backdrop, individual agency means to know how to maintain a certain degree of independence by utilising body-knowledge, experiential knowledge, and social assertiveness, all of which are informed by and entangled with medical lay-expertise. This enables persons with IBD to not only interact in acute illness phases with their social world (e.g. family members, co-workers) but also to become actionable while gaining the ability to contextualise and evaluate the explanations given to them by medical experts. Such patients can be best described as their own experts at the intersection between living a disease/condition and a disease/condition as a medico-scientific object (Willhelm et al. 2015).

Autonomy and the Limitations of the Health Platform Economy

By making use of the infrastructures provided by social health networks, some groups of users enable themselves not only to discuss treatment options, share medical advice, co-create data, and illness-narratives but also to form emergent concerned collectives (Callon and Rabeharisoa 2007).

A very recent example for such collectives is the self-organisation and the scientifico-political activity of feminist health-groups on PatientsLikeMe. In spring 2017, against the backdrop of a worldwide backlash against women's reproductive rights. This backlash was connected to the rise of a new right wing conservatism around the globe, including South-America, the United States, and various European countries (see P8_TA(2019)0111). Subsequently, discussions about cycle studies and methods like menstrual extraction (see Chap. 4 of this book) began to trend in the network's research forums. Both young women and seasoned self-help veterans began to share their first-hand knowledge about bodily autonomy, to reflect the socio-historical developments of their experiences within the healthcare-system, and began to form both political and lay-research alliances to find a modern approach to decolonise women's bodies. This is remarkable because of the fact that decades after the legalisation and normalisation of abortion in many states around the world, such discussions and practices seem to become necessary once more. In addition, involvement also bridges a generational gap of activism and responsibilities in "women's sisterhood", and further emphasises the strengths and limitations of grassroots feminist activism in data-centred (semi-)commercial social health networks.

The conflicted relationship between alternative approaches and related techniques of the body and its institutionalised counterparts marks the limitations for the participation of activists and other personally concerned individuals who seek to co-produce and disseminate their experiential knowledge in social health networks. This can be observed especially when they challenge common beliefs and the implicit moralities of a society reflected in the network. In short, this tension can be noted when participants/users cross the boundaries of the dominant political discourse. The tension became evident in spring of 2017, when the discussion about menstrual extraction on the PatiensLikeMe platform became politicised by some users (like the professionals in the 1970s), who re-framed it as a risky and an illegal abortion method. Ultimately, the topic "menstrual extraction" disappeared from the network (see PLM discussion "harpgirl" ME 2012). Whether this disappearance is due to political agitation by critical users, or due to the implicit morality of the network itself remains unclear. Consequentially, this episode underscores the moralised boundaries and implicit restrictions of both semi-commercial and fully commercialised health-networks. They are not a place for countercultural experimentation or knowledge dissemination with respect to health practices but are operating tightly within the confines of the status quo. This is evidenced, when they, like in the case of menstrual extraction, might increase the options of concerned and oftentimes marginalised individuals. It is noteworthy that DIY-practices like menstrual extraction are re-emerging not only as elements of a certain lifestyle (i.e. educated middle-class populations) but also as a necessity for those who are losing the opportunity for bodily autonomy within an increasingly re-moralised and austerised health-care culture.

3.3 Sense-Making

Individuals suffering from Crohn's disease or ulcerative colitis are also beginning to discuss DIY-practices to increase their bodily autonomy. While not framed as politically sensitive as menstrual extraction, they are nevertheless beyond the governmental epistemological framing of both institutionalised medicine and the codes of conduct of most participatory social health platforms. This is especially true in the area faecal transplantations. Where discussions are constantly crossing the boundaries between accepted medical practice and potentially harmful self-medication. Therefore, they might become in the future also practices "non grata".

The microbiome of the gut has become in recent years not only a hot topic in research about immune processes and inflammation, but also a focal point for popular science media (see Mahr 2017). It is, therefore, not surprising that individuals with Crohn's disease or ulcerative colitis are hopeful with regard to the possibility of influencing the composition of their gut microbes in a way that might have a positive impact on their condition. Unlike the genetic explanation of their condition, which can be understood by some as fate, they associate with the microbiome an increased level of health-related agency. It enables them to participate in health or medical settings with the aim of gaining a higher degree of sovereignty over their own bodies or to alter the public perception of their bodies and experiences. This can go hand in hand with the acquisition of individual options for action or influence, whether in an individual's social life, the political sphere, or with respect to the medico-scientific system.

A look at social health networks like PatiensLikeMe or other Web 2.0 self-help structures seems to confirm this. There, individuals with chronic inflammatory bowel disorders are excitedly discussing how the microbiome approach could help them with their condition. Many of them are particularly interested in the practices and offers that are also highlighted in the media discourse about the microbiome: stool-donations for research projects such as Britishgut, the offers of commercial direct-to-consumer sequencing providers and the DIY culture surrounding faecal transplantation. Three forms of action are discussed: participation in research that seeks to discover the causes for inflammatory intestinal diseases (1), the usability of knowledge about the composition of one's own microbiome for the improvement of individual intestinal health (2), and how to replace one's own microbiome with that of a person without chronic inflammatory bowel diseases (3). At the end of 2014, the practice of stool transplantation was lively discussed in the forum of the German Crohn's Disease/Ulcerative Colitis. A user suffering from ulcerative colitis raised the topic and asked in the forum how she could carry out a transplant in Germany or Europe. In practice, this project might sound "disgusting" (…), but "somehow she also thinks" (…): "I have nothing to lose" (…) (DCCV Forum 11/2014). A regular user in the forum – User B – replied that there are various clinical studies, but stated that the practice is still highly controversial. The US Food and Drug Administration (FDA), for example, only allows them in special cases (see Young 2014). His look at American health networks and forums, where study participants shared their experiences with other sufferers, showed that "there are 50% remission rates for ulcerative colitis (…)" (Young 2014). This also fits into the picture of a new research study that says that transplantation is also successful in some forms of colitis. He refers to a study by Atarashi K. et al. with the title "Induction of colonic regulatory T cells by indigenous Clostridium species", that refers to success, but is limited to a mouse model (Atarashi et al. 2011). User B also points out that only two medical practitioners in Hamburg and Zurich are offering a transplant in Europe so far. He therefore advises the creator of the thread to get more information on the website thepowerofpoop.com, which is a portal that provides information on how faecal transplants are performed by doctors, that disseminates information about ongoing studies as well as instructions for stool transplantation at home (The Power of Poop 2016). Another user, C, complements B's contribution and states that there are already a few "short publications of FMT/stool transplants within Germany and Switzerland (available) (…), for example the ones conducted at the Kurpfalzkrankenhaus in Heidelberg, (…) at the Hospital in Bremen or another one at the University Clinic of Jena" (DCCV-Forum 2014). But he also points out that most clinics in German-speaking countries predominantly seek to treat Clostridium difficile but that some private practitioners might be "more open for experiments" (Ibid.). Therefore, the "IBD community" in Germany would be eager to receive information about how this form of therapy could be beneficial for the treatment of ulcerative colitis or even Crohn's disease (Ibid.). A short time after this post, another user, D, who appears to be active also within the PatientLikeMe community and uses the forum of thepowerofpoop. com frequently, posts the following statement:

> Hi, I'm going to start a self-experiment in the next few weeks according to the DIY instructions. I have CD [Crohn's disease – the author] (…) but it's worth a try. The effort is low and so is the cost. On Thursday I have an appointment with my gastro(enterologist – the author) who tests the donor (blood and stool sample). As soon as the results are received, I start the transplant. At the beginning of March I had an appointment with another gastroenterologist who answered the following to my question about the FMT (fecal transplantation – the author): 'Dear Sir *****, we can do it, but then as a private service. But you would have to introduce yourself first to a preliminary discussion.' The doctor already has experience in the treatment of C.difficile with FMT. If there is interest, I can briefly report on how things are going with me. (DCCV-Forum 2014)

The announcement of a self-experiment accompanied by a doctor generates further discussion in the forum. Two positions are dominant. Firstly, there are people who point out the lack of evidence of scientific evidence for success in Crohn's disease, and who are also sceptical about the safety of the procedure (contamination, infections, etc.). The vast majority of forum participants, however, is very open and interested. Most are looking forward to an experience report from "the first stool-transplant user within the community". User D is also asked about who would provide the donation. He replies to this question that his mother is providing the stool and that he is aware about the lack of scientific evidence of Crohn's disease. However, he argues, that he has also read some positive case reports on the international patient platform healingwell.com.

This short excerpt from a German-speaking community for people with inflammatory bowel diseases illustrates how affected individuals make sense out of both their condition and the scientific discourse & practices surrounding it, in order to gain agency. Their main tools seem to be both the utilisation of online information and networked communities of individuals with similar experiences as well as the transfer of shared knowledge into their own bodily practices of the self which include self-experimentation. The online organised IBD patients are well informed about scientific developments but are also self-confident experts of their own illness experiences. Their activities are oscillating between the sphere of online activity and real-life actionability. For them, the emergence of social health networks seems to be highly beneficial. But the question remains: Are they aware of the extent of personal health information they are disclosing publicly?

3.4   The Dilemma of Data

While the idealisation of the individual signifies a retribution of responsibilities from the state to the individual member of society, its customisation emphasises the identity aspect of choice. Against the backdrop of my socio-economic or cultural status, I am able to make health related choices, for example, about insurance plans, nutritional habits, forms and frequency of exercise, medical professionals, and most recently also about with whom I want to share my health-information. It is not only a question of if I want to share my health information with others (be it for the purpose of comparison, to get/give advice, or to contribute to research) but also a question of where to share the information. Therefore, I as an individual am held (prospectively) responsible for the choice of a platform and ultimately for the use and re-use of my information by third parties. The moral foundation of personalised health, as such reveals its core flaw: The implicit force for self-care, responsibility and choice will result in dilemmas, specifically, am I willing to give up a certain part of my informational identity in order to fully meet the inherent demand for health-related self-care and informational altruism?

A growing number individuals suffering from chronic inflammatory bowel diseases are confronted with such aforementioned dilemmas. Whether they seek a community with similar experiences, want to contribute to research via self-reporting on PatiensLikeMe, specialised platforms like Crohnology, or turn to (less well known) non-commercial alternatives, they are unconsciously making a responsibility-choice to give up control over their information. They do so in exchange for access to a community that promises them more agency in navigating their condition and to better the lives of others as well. How this kind of "donating data for individual and collective agency" shall work is clearly displayed on the starting page of crohnology.com. Here, the providers describe the perks of self-governance and self-reporting and how the produced information will be looped back into the community. Furthermore, they show how deeply they epistemologically believe in quantification, since they count the number of affected individuals who have subscribed to their services, the countries they are coming from and the "years of patient experience" they have so far collected (crohnology.com 2020) (see Fig. 3.3).

There are currently over 11,000 subscribers on Crohnology and about 2000 of them are sharing their treatments, dietary experiences and other information on a regular basis. However, three years ago some individuals of its community grew sceptical towards both the claims of self-improvement through public self-management and the data practices of social health networks. This might be either informed by a raised awareness for health related data security in recent years (see Casola et al. 2016) or due to a digital divide within the user base of the network. A good argument for the latter is the fact that those who express their scepticism are additionally active on self-governed infrastructures (such as the

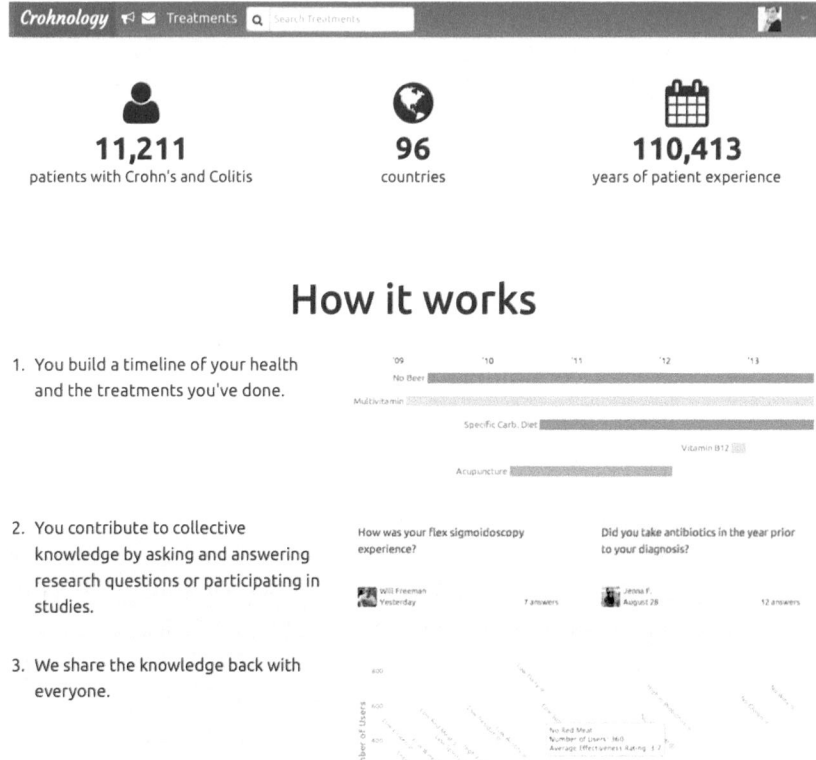

Fig. 3.3 Crohnology.com (2020)

Crohn's community on Reddit or related chat-rooms on discord), pre-dominantly frequented by tech-savvy individuals. An example for this critical engagement is the thread "Crohn's knowledge sharing website" on r/CrohnsDisease (2017).

The creator of the post (user A) introduces himself as someone who was diagnosed with Crohn's disease in the year 2014 while studying computer science in college. He further discloses that he is planning to set up a new resource for sharing experiences and knowledge about the condition:

> I am setting up a website that allows Crohn's sufferers to pool together their knowledge. Forums, and this subreddit, provide a great resource for getting answers to your questions, but there is poor search functionality for old threads, and importantly, little to distinguish quality answers from unhelpful answers. The karma system on Reddit goes some way towards this, but I believe that a tailor-made solution would be better.
>
> I have two distinct formats:
>
> 1. A Wikipedia style website, where contributions center around specific topics – pages for stoma care, diets, typical treatment pathways, surgeries etc....
> 2. A question and answer website, rewarding approved contributors (like StackOverflow), with a great search function. This prevents contributors answering the same questions multiple times, and the spreading of misinformation.
>
> Let me know your thoughts on these two options, and the concept. Which would you find useful? What would encourage you to contribute on a different website? (r/Crohnsdisease 2017)

In the following discussion another person, user B, points out her/his/their experience with and opinion about the aforementioned website Crohnology:

> I have – Crohnology is designed to harvest profitable datasets from users. I hate that to access the information you have to create an account – that totally goes against my goal of instantly accessible, legible information for sufferers. Do you use Crohnology? (r/Crohnsdisease 2017)

In her/his/their commentary, user B, shows not only understanding about the business practices and goals of commercial or semi-commercial social health networks, but also criticises that information on such platforms as bound to the creation of an user account. It's apparent that this user is also technology savvy and prefers open information and anonymity over the common practice of membership. In his answer to this statement user A writes, that he doesn't use the platform, "partly for the data collection aspect" (r/Crohnsdisease 2017). Another user, C adds to the discussion the point, that a "properly maintained" question and answer section "would be great because there are always things that aren't posted on pubmed or the national library of medicine pages for Crohn's issues" (Ibid.).

Another example is user D, who discussed in the sub forum "Bearableapp" with other users about what a "mood & symptom tracking app" for them should include and how it should deal with privacy. The beta result (which user D introduced finally in November 2019) then, takes into account, that plenty of knowledge about such conditions has a highly individual character. Therefore, it allows users to develop, while using the app, their own system of categories and to make use of a diary function. Furthermore, according to D, it is written to be an application that is fully operational without sharing any data with the developers while shared information will not be used in any commercial setting.

This brief insight into the Crohn's and colitis community active on Reddit shows that a relatively large number of patients have an intrinsic commitment to make information accessible to one another. They are therefore looking for valid and helpful information that is not hidden behind either a paywall or has to be bought at the cost of a (partly forced) disclosure of private information. Instead they are actively generating their own form of agency within the hybrid world of informational technology, corporate interests, and societal enforced self-care by engaging with the spirit of the early years of the internet. But even beyond this reinforcement of the open source and anonymity ethos of the "old" internet, there is something different about this part of the community of people with chronic inflammatory bowel diseases; this difference being one of epistemological nature. In contrast to what is presented as "patient experience" on platforms like PatientsLikeMe, where the experiential knowledge expressed within individual illness narratives is either regarded as a marginal secondary source or gets outright devalued in favour of quantifiable information, narratives of living with a condition like Crohn's or colitis receives encouragement by the r/Crohnsdisease community. There are hundreds of threads in which individuals share very sensitive and private information about themselves; share thoughts, compare their experiences, comfort each other, and discuss ways in which they could better their situations (r/Crohnsdisease 2020; see: r/IAmA 2012). Thus, a minority population within the community of people suffering from Crohn's disease and ulcerative colitis seeks to develop their own tools and practices to deal with the inherent data dilemmas that are connected to self-care in data-centered societies and their (in terms of privacy) ambivalent operating healthcare systems.

Even if the general trend of the development of the self-help culture goes in the direction of formalisation, commercialisation and centralisation of a few commercial and semi-commercial platforms, there are also indications in increased form that some users give a change to non-commercial alternatives that do not violate the data privacy. Examples for this are new inclusive health movements that seek to transcend the offline-online boundary. Proponents of the DIY culture and alternative health platforms begin to combine health information and activism with artistic expression. Examples include the Open Source Estrogen Project (Tsang 2020), the Open Insulin Project (Smith 2019), the revival of the Gimp Girl Community (Cole et al. 2011) for women with physical disabilities, and various queer-feminist and intersectional health collectives (Mahr and Prüll 2018).

3.5 Conclusion

In this chapter I analysed three levels of interconnection between social health platforms, their users, the health care system, and the medical sciences: The digitalisation of self-help culture, the various ambiguities of this process, and how patients/users develop resilience towards the economic and political implications of its data oriented understanding of health.

During the 1980s and 1990s many individuals with chronic illnesses had to face the social and medical challenges of their illness in limited and sometimes isolating conditions. Today's healthcare culture, in contrast, challenges them to navigate through an overabundance of incentives to participate and societal expectations to care about themselves. Ever since austerity became one of the driving forces in western healthcare systems during the 2010s, the paradigm of personalised health has gained momentum. Under the umbrella of this concept, prevention and participation evolved into core values asking those who suffer from certain conditions (or might have a "risk" to develop them) to become proactive actors with regard to their own health. This form of self-care has little to do with the self-governed and bottom-up organised health activism of the 1970s, despite the fact that some actors like governments or the health care industry invoke similar terminology in their campaigns and advertisements today. In the past, self-care meant emancipation of marginalised groups such as the LGBTQIA+ community during the HIV-crisis. Oftentimes, it was connected to alternative epistemilac and practical approaches towards medicine and its institutions. Today's mainstream self-care aims to maintain given assumptions and ideas about health, illness, and their underlying politics albeit in a condensed quantifiable form. This maintaining of the status quo becomes apparent when analysing the shared boundaries between the medical sciences, the healthcare sector, and exponents of the modern data economy. The relationship towards the latter remains for some national actors ambiguous primarily due to questions about data security and ownership. However, its quantified approach towards health seems to be highly compatible with recent understandings of individual self-care within the paradigm of personalised health. Against this backdrop slogans like "Donate your data for you, for others, for good" (PatientsLikeMe), "What if we could learn from the collective experience of patients everywhere?" (Crohnicity) or "What can be done to make the health system more sustainable?" (Swiss Personalized Health Network 2020) gain meaning and power.

Health care in the twenty-first century requires an individual commitment to self-help. Commercial online patient networks offer this, but at the price of the disclosure of the self in the form of a data donation. Many patients take the commitment to self-help seriously and seek community and information about their own disease on platforms such as PatientsLikeMe, Ben's Friends, or CureTogether. They rationalise this as a responsibility towards themselves, their families and the society in which they live. However, given the fact that our society and politics are (still) ambivalent on the issue of disclosure of personal health information towards third parties, users of online health networks are faced with a dilemma. This dilemma is one which, against the background of the datafication of all areas of life and knowledge, also (paradoxically) forms the business basis of such networks. This also seems to be one of the reasons why many of these platforms are rather conservative in terms of health epistemology. They do not want to alienate research institutions and state actors as potential customers, even when they criticise them rhetorically. The dilemma of disclosure of personal health information along with the strategic, epistemic and political conservatism of participatory social health networks have led some potential users to look for alternative forms of digital self-help in the online context.

Examples of these alternatives are the various DIY forums in which people suffering from Crohn's disease or ulcerative colitis discuss and test alternative treatment regimes. At the moment the focus is on faecal transplantation which is not approved by the FDA. The subject, therefore, is a potentially problematic one for these patients and is therefore potentially problematic to discuss on networks such as PatientsLikeMe. The users who are active in these DIY forums find agency in looking for help and experimenting with new things beyond the health system's restrictions. Their empowerment consists in testing epistemic diversity. A different approach is taken by all those who accept the data logic of the health care system and networks. Such individuals seek to monitor and share their own health in a quantified form, but are simultaneously sceptical about the public release and potential loss of ownership of their health data. For this particular group, agency means that they can handle their information in a self-determined way. In the forum r/Crohnsdisease and on the platform OpenSNP such participants find a platform.

However, the question remains: What has become of Nico and his mother? In short, they report not to feel isolated anymore. Nico's mother established an account on PatientsLikeMe five years ago. She intends to experiment with DIY-faecal transplantation. The community, she says, "will not only help her to find a medical practitioner to assist her in this journey", but also has agreed to support her through all of her journey.

For this, she plans to upload a live video-blog on YouTube. Nico has since become an IT-expert. He seems to be a bit more concerned about the use of PatientsLikeMe, especially with regards to the data security. Nevertheless, when last I met him in my hometown, he told me that he is relieved that there has been much advancement in the last two decades. This he believes has been possible primarily due to the online self-help structures.

References

Atarashi, Koji, Takeshi Tanoue, Tatsuichiro Shima, Akemi Imaoka, Tomomi Kuwahara, Yoshika Momose, Genhong Cheng, Sho Yamasaki, Takashi Saito, Yusuke Ohba, Tadatsugu Taniguchi, Kiyoshi Takeda, Shohei Hori, Ivaylo I. Ivanov, Yoshinori Umesaki, Kikuji Ithoh, and Keny Honda. 2011. Induction of Colonic Regulatory T Cells by Indigenous Clostridium Species. *Science* 331 (6015): 337–341. https://doi.org/10.1126/science.1198469. Accessed 6 Apr 2020.

Banner, Olivia. 2017. *Communicative Biocapitalism*. Arbor: Michigan Publishing.

Benkler, Yochai. 2006. *The Wealth of Networks: How Social Production Transforms Markets and Freedom*. New Haven: Yale University Press.

Callon, Michel, and Rabeharisoa Vololona. 2007. The Growing Engagement of Emergent Concerned Groups in Political and Economic Life: Lessons from the French Association of Neuromuscular Disease Patients. *Science, Technology, & Human Values* 33 (2): 230–261.

Casilli, Antonio A., and Julian Posada Gutierrez. 2019. The Platformization of Labor and Society. In *Society and the Internet*, ed. M. Graham and W.H. Dutton, 2nd ed., 293–306. Oxford University Press.

Casola, Valentina, Aniello Castiglione, Raymond Choo Kim-Kwang, and Christian Esposito. 2016. *Healthcare-Related Data in the Cloud: Challenges and Opportunities*. https://doi.org/10.1109/MCC.2016.139. Accessed 9 Dec 2020.

Chateuvert, Melinda. 2013. *Sex Workers Unite. A History of the Movement from Stonewall to Slut Walk*. Boston: Beacon Press.

Cole, Jennifer, Jason Nolan, Yukari Seko, Katherine Mancuso, and Alejandra Ospina. 2011. GimpGirl Grows Up: Women with Disabilities Rethinking, Redefining, and Reclaiming Community. *New Media & Society* 13 (7): 1161–1179.

Conrad, Peter, and Cheryl Stults. 2010. The Internet and the Experience of Illness. In *Handbook of Medical Sociology*, 179–191. Nashville: Vanderbilt University Press.

Crohn's and Colitis UK. 2015. *Crohn's and Colitis Awareness.*https://www.facebook.com/CrohnsColitisAwareness/posts/890843521000986. Accessed 9 Dec 2020.

Crohnology. 2020. https://crohnology.com/. Accessed 9 Dec 2020.

DCCV-Forum. 2014. *Thema Genetik.* https://forum.dccv.de/viewtopic.php?f=3&t=1806. Accessed 9 Dec 2020.

Epstein, Steven. 1995. The Construction of Lay Expertise: AIDS Activism and the Forging of Credibility in the Reform of Clinical Trials. *Science, Technology, & Human Values* 20 (4): 408–437.

FFWHC – Federation of Feminist Women's Health Centers. 1991. *A New View of a Woman's Body. A Fully Illustrated Guide.* 10th anniversary ed. West Hollywood: Feminist Health Press.

Foucault, Michel, and Gordon Colin. 1980. *Power/Knowledge: Selected Interviews and Other Writings 1972–1977.* New York: Vintage Books.

Frankfort, Ellen. 1973. Medicine, the Feminist Frontier. *The New York Times*, March 3.

Garcia-Sanjuan, Sofia, Manuel Lillo-Crespo, Angela Sanjuan-Quiles, Diana Gil-Gonzales, and Miguel Richart-Martinez. 2016. Life Experiences of People Affected by Crohn's Disease and Their Support Networks: Scoping Review. *Clinical Nursing Research* 25 (1): 79–99.

Greshake Tzovaras, Bastian. 2020. *E-Mail – Bastian Greshake Tzovaras and Dana Mahr*, January 7. https://outlook.unige.ch/owa/#path=/mail. Accessed 9 Dec 2020.

Grosberg, Dafna, Haya Grinvald, Haim Reuveni, and Racheli Magnezi. 2016. Frequent Surfing on Social Health Networks is Associated with Increased Knowledge and Patient Health Activation. *Journal of Medical Internet Research* 18 (8). https://doi.org/10.2196/jmir.5832. Accessed 9 Dec 2020.

harpgirl. 2012. Menstrual Extractions: Controversy and Safety. *Social Health Network. Political Mingling (PLM Forum)*, August 24. https://www.patientslikeme.com/forum/ms/topics/102276?post_id=1759024#post-1759024. Accessed 9 Dec 2020.

Heffernan, Virginia. 2011. Online Medical Advice Can Be a Prescription for Fear. *The New York Times*, February 4, sec. Magazine. https://www.nytimes.com/2011/02/06/magazine/06FOB-Medium-t.html. Accessed 9 Dec 2020.

Hoffman, Lily M. 1982. *The Politics of Knowledge. Activist Movements in Medicine and Planning.* New York: State University of New York Press.

Høivik, Marte Lee, Tomm Bernklev, Inger Camilla Solberg, Milada Cvancarova, Ida Lygren, Jørgen Jahnsen, and Bjørn Moum. 2012. The IBSEN Study Group, Patients with Crohn's Disease Experience Reduced General Health and Vitality in the Chronic Stage: Ten-Year Results from the IBSEN Study. *Journal of Crohn's and Colitis* 6 (4): 441–453. https://doi.org/10.1016/j.crohns.2011.10.001. Accessed 18 Dec 2020.

Huh, Jina, Rebecca Marmor, and Xiaoqian Jiang. 2016. Lessons Learned for Online Health Community Moderator Roles: A Mixed-Methods Study of Moderators Resigning from WebMD Communities. *Journal of Medical Internet Research* 18 (9): e247. https://doi.org/10.2196/jmir.6331. Accessed 18 Dec 2020.

Janssens, A., J.W. Cecile, and Peter Kraft. 2012. Research Conducted Using Data Obtained Through Online Communities: Ethical Implications of Methodological Limitations. *PloS Med* 9 (10): e1001328.

Kalafateli, Maria, Christos Triantos, Georgios Theocharis, Dimitra Giannakopoulou, Efstratios Koutroumpakis, Chronis Aristidis, Apostolos Sapountzis Vasileios Margaritis, Konstantinos Thomopoulos, and Vasiliki Nikolopoulou. 2013. Health-Related Quality of Life in Patients with Inflammatory Bowel Disease: A Single-Center Experience. *Annals of Gastroenterology* 26 (3): 243–248.

Katrini, Eleni. 2018. Sharing Culture: On Definitions, Values, and Emergence. *The Sociological Review* 66 (2): 425–446. https://doi.org/10.1177/0038026118758550. Accessed 18 Dec 2020.

Lupton, Deborah. 2014. The Commodification of Patient Opinion: The Digital Patient Experience Economy in the Age of Big Data. *Sociology of Health & Illness* 36 (6). https://doi.org/10.1111/1467-9566.12109. Accessed 18 Dec 2020.

Magnezi, Racheli, Yoav S. Bergman, and Dafna Grosberg. 2014. Online Activity and Participation in Treatment Affects the Perceived Efficacy of Social Health Networks Among Patients with Chronic Illness. *Journal of Medical Internet Research* 16 (1). https://doi.org/10.2196/jmir.2630. Accessed 18 Dec 2020.

Mahr, Dana. 2017. Self-Reporting and Participatory Health Platforms: Empowerment Through Sharing Information About Onself Online? *Harvard Bill of Health*. https://blog.petrieflom.law.harvard.edu/2017/05/01/self-reporting-and-participatory-health-platforms-empowerment-through-sharing-information-about-oneself-online/. Accessed 18 Dec 2020.

Mahr, Dana, and Livia Prüll. 2018. Körperliche Selbstermächtigung aus dem 3D-Drucker? Feministische Kulturen als Parallelwelten und der Kampf um gesellschaftliche Teilhabe seit 1970. In *Kybernetik, Kapitalismus, Revolutionen.*

Emanzipatorische Perspektiven im technologischen Wandel, ed. Paul Buckermann, Anne Koppenburg, and Simon Schaub, 161–190. Münster: Unrast.

Mahr, Dana, Eva Mahr, and Christoph Rehmann-Sutter. 2019. Subjektivierungsfiguren Genetischer Information. *Sozialer Sinn* 20 (1): 1–39. https://doi.org/10.1515/sosi-2019-0001. Accessed 18 Dec 2020.

Martinez, Bibiana, Francis Dailey, Christopher V. Almario, Michelle S. Keller, Mansee Desai, Taylor Dupuy, Sasan Mosadeghi, Cynthia Whitman, Karen Lasch, Lyann Ursos, and Brennan M.R. Spiegel. 2017. Patient Understanding of the Risks and Benefits of Biologic Therapies in Inflammatory Bowel Disease: Insights from a Large-Scale Analysis of Social Media Platforms. *Inflammatory Bowel Diseases* 23 (7): 1057–1064.

Moran, Rachel Louise. 2018. *Governing Bodies. American Politics and the Shaping of the Modern Physique*. Philadelphia: University of Pennsylvania Press.

Morgen, Sandra. 2002. *Into Our Own Hands: The Women's Health Movement in the United States, 1969–1990*. New Brunswick: Rutgers University Press.

Neal, Lisa, Gitte Lindgaard, Kate Oakley, Derek Hansen, Sandra Kogan, Jan Marco Leimeister, Ted Selker. 2006. "Online Health Communities" 'CHI' 06. *Extended Abstracts on Human Factors in Computing Systems*, 444–447. New York: Association for Computing Machinery. https://doi.org/10.1145/1125451.1125549. Accessed 18 Dec 2020.

Nelson, Alondra. 2011. *Body and Soul. The Black Panther Party and the Fight Against Medical Discrimination*. Minneapolis: University of Minnesota Press.

O'Neil, Cathy. 2016. *Weapons of Math Destruction. How Big Data Increases Inequality and Threatens Democracy*. London: Penguin Books.

OpenSNP. 2020. *FAQ*. https://opensnp.org/faq. Accessed 18 Dec 2020.

PatientsLikeMe. 2016. *Blog: Data for Good*. https://blog.patientslikeme.com/a-new-year-a-new-goal/. Accessed 25 July 2021.

———. 2020. *Overview PLM*. https://www.patientslikeme.com/. Accessed 18 Dec 2020.

Porter, Theodore M. 1995. *Trust in Numbers. The Pursuit of Objectivity in Science and Public Life*. Princeton: Princeton University Press.

Prainsack, Barbara. 2014. The Powers of Participatory Medicine. *PLoS Biology* 12 (4): e1001837. Accessed 18 Dec 2020.

———. 2020. Data Mining in Systems Medicine and the Project of Solidarity: The Interface of Genomics and Society Revisited. In *De-Sequencing. Identity Work with Genes*, ed. Dana Mahr and Martina von Arx, 97–117. Basingstoke: Palgrave Macmillan.

Prainsack, Barbara, and Alena Buyx. 2017. *Solidarity in Biomedicine and Beyond.* Cambridge: Cambridge University Press.

reddit. 2017. *R/CrohnsDisease.* https://www.reddit.com/r/CrohnsDisease/. Accessed 18 Dec 2020.

———. 2020. *R/CrohnsDisease.* https://www.reddit.com/r/CrohnsDisease/. Accessed 18 Dec 2020.

Reddit r/IAmA. 2012. *Crohn's Experience.* https://www.reddit.com/r/IAmA/. Accessed 25 July 2021.

Rochelle, Tina L., and Helen Fidler. 2012. The Importance of Illness Perceptions, Quality of Life and Psychological Status in Patients with Ulcerative Colitis and Crohn's Disease. *Journal of Health Psychology* 18 (7): 972–983.

Smith, Dana G. 2019. Biohackers with Diabetes Are Making Their Own Insulin. *Medium* (online). https://elemental.medium.com/biohackers-with-diabetes-are-making-their-own-insulin-edbfbea8386d. Accessed 18 Dec 2020.

Strasser, Bruno, Jerome Baudry, Dana Mahr, Gabriela Sanchez, and Elise Tancoigne. 2019. Citizen Science? Rethinking Science and Public Participation. *Science & Technology Studies* 32 (2): 52–76.

Stuckler, David, and Sanjay Basu. 2013. *The Body Economic. Why Austerity Kills.* New York: Basic Books.

Swiss Personalized Health Network (SPHN). 2020. *Infrastructure Building to Enable Nationwide Use and Exchange of Health Data for Research.* https://sphn.ch/. Accessed 25 July 2021.

Tempini, Niccolo. 2014. PatientsLikeMe.com: Developing Medical Research from Social Data. *LSE Research Festival 2014*, 2014-05-08. http://eprints.lse.ac.uk/57927/. Accessed 18 Dec 2020.

The Power of Poop. 2016. *The Power of Poop | Promoting Safe Accessible Fecal Transplant.* http://thepowerofpoop.com/. Accessed 18 Dec 2020.

Tsang, Mary. 2020. *Open Source Estrogen. Housewives Making Drugs.* https://www.media.mit.edu/projects/open-source-estrogen/overview/. Accessed 18 Dec 2020.

Weinberger, David. 2012. *Too Big to Know: Rethinking Knowledge Now that the Facts Aren't the Facts, Experts Are Everywhere, and the Smartest Person in the Room Is the Room.* New York: Basic Books.

Wicks, Paul, Timothy E. Vaughan, Michael P. Massagli, and James Heywood. 2011. Accelerated Clinical Discovery Using Self-Reported Patient Data Collected Online and a Patient-Matching Algorithm. *Nature Biotechnology* 29 (5): 411–414. Accessed 18 Dec 2020.

Wilburn, Jeanette, James Twiss, Karen Kemp, and Stephen P. McKenna. 2017. A Qualitative Study of the Impact of Crohn's Disease from a Patient's

Perspective. *Frontline Gastroenterology* 8 (1): 68–73. https://doi.org/10.1136/flgastro-2015-100678. Accessed 18 Dec 2020.

Wilhelm, Nadja, and Dana (geb. Dominik) Mahr, and Christoph Rehmann-Sutter. 2015. Stoma als Wende. *Bauchredner* 1: 8.

Willis, Erin, and Marla B. Royne. 2017. Online Health Communities and Chronic Dsiease Self-Management. *Health Communication* 32: 269–278.

Yom-Tov, Elad. 2016. *Crowdsourced Health: How What You Do on the Internet Will Improve Medicine*. Cambridge: MIT Press.

Young, Kenneth A. 2014. Of Poop and Parasites: Unethical FDA Overregulation. *Food & Drug Law Journal* 69: 555–563.

4

Radical Feminist Movements and the Re-Imagination of Performative Epistemology

Abstract This chapter explores new forms of intersectional and body-related, partially performative feminism that emerges in the current socio-political climate. Hence the neo-conservative climate in many parts of the world threatens to curtail women's rights once again. New feminist movements are, on the one hand, rediscovering the body-related practices of the 1960s. However, on the other hand, they enrich them with new epistemic and social values such as "sharing possibilities", "applicability to human needs", and "intercultural sensitivity". This creates a new form of knowledge production that, for example, pushes the boundaries between art, politics, and science and transcends reductionist understandings of epistemic activities.

Keywords Performativity • DIY health • Women's health movement • Values in science

In August 2014, activists of the so-called GynePunk movement met in Calafou (Barcelona), a post-capitalist commune, for the first international TransHackFeminist Convergence. The goal of this meeting was to bring together feminists, trans* and queer people of all genders to exchange, understand and develop new accessible and liberating technologies for the advancement of social participation in health for marginalised people (Colonia ecoindustrial postcapitalista 2014). This included gender hacking with self-produced hormone therapies, experiments with gynaecological self-examination with open-source tools, and the creation of instructions for the identification and DIY treatment of sexually transmittable diseases in simple language. All the know-how produced during this workshop focused on a social goal: to expand access to reproductive health care and reconfigure it in a participatory way, placing special emphasis on groups like sex workers and (illegal) immigrants.

The GynePunk movement frames such activities as a way to appropriate existing and explore new medical technologies from an alternative epistemological angle: open health for human needs instead of medical paternalism and exclusion of those who can't afford or can't access dignified healthcare. In parallel, such activities align with the aesthetics and values of bio-technological avant-garde movements like that of biohackers and makers. Accordingly, the GynePunks communicate their actions in the mode of the unprecedented, counter-cultural and revolutionary (Lewis 2006; Wohlsen 2011; Jen 2015). For example, in an interview with the former WIRED journalist Dough Bierend, the GynePunk activist Klau Kinky characterises the identity of the movement as follows: "The (…) criteria I would apply to consider yourself GynePunk is reclaiming your body" (Bierend 2015).

But is the motif of reclaiming one's own body really as closely linked to the rejection of current forms of medical governmentally and the capitalist economy as their activists' rhetoric suggests? How dependent is their culture of technically induced participation on web-based communication technologies, and alternative forms of ownership such as open-source or creative commons? Is the activism of the GynePunks part of a historical tradition – and if so: how does this change our view on health activism and epistemic diversity in the early twenty-first century?

In this chapter I would like explore some possible answers to this question. First, I will place the project of the GynePunks into a broader sociohistorical context. Specifically, I will discuss how people who are considered as "different" by the wider public and who are in need of medical services negotiate with both the epistemic and political institutions of medicine. In the following section, I look at the GynePunks themselves and proceed asynchronously in a comparative manner: I compare the activism and knowledge culture of the GynePunk Movement with that of the early Women's Health Movement of the 1970s. In doing so, I not only look for intersections, differences and traditions on the level of concrete practice, but also try to gain a perspective on their engagements with knowledge institutions. I also investigate the socio-economic, political, and epistemic conditions that influence both in the counter cultural movements of the 1960s and today to self-empowering health movements.

4.1 "Other" People and Social "Parallel Worlds"

When asked what the GynePunks actually represent, one is inevitably challenged to make fundamental considerations. These considerations concern the relationship of people to scientific medicine and its representatives. The question of how people can come to terms with medical topics, theories, measures and instructions in very special cases becomes a persistent one. If we take this step, we will be able to classify the GynePunks with their special concerns.

First of all, it must be noted that in Western Europe and the USA, scientific medicine succeeded around 1850 in maintaining the power of interpretation with respect to questions of health and illness (Labisch 1991). With the help of repeatable and controlled experiments within the framework of an unbiased perceived view of nature, an effectiveness could be demonstrated that made scientific medicine (as one approach among many) finally the "orthodox medicine" (Bynum 1994; Bynum et al. 2006). This initially implied that other approaches, which were then labelled as "alternative medicine", receded into the background. More importantly, in our context, however, is that in the special situation of the nineteenth century, the representatives of scientific medicine fought for the authorisation to let their expertise become socio-politically effective in an extraordinary way. Not only did the influence of medical parameters and facts on various social groups increase, but this influence went further and took a breathtaking step towards a health-political screening of society. This was done by coupling the morphological substrate of its population into a "sick" and a "healthy" state both behaviourally and bodily. The task was to standardise the groups in society and then identify, define, and regulate those which did not conform to the given normative concepts.

The Darwinian theory of descendancy also provided the aforementioned procedure with a heuristic matrix. According to these views, the coupling of deviant physicality and deviant social behaviour was caused by degenerated genetic material. Its carriers were thus definitely stigmatised (Planert 2000). It is now remarkable that this by no means affected only those groups that we now call "patients" in our perception. It is true that psychiatric patients in particular, along with "syphilitics", "alcoholics", and others, were known to have been targeted by medical investigators for "abnormality". But, there were also groups that simply attracted attention because of their social behaviour and were caught in the spell of medical care and prevention within the context of pathologisation. They thought they could recognise criminals by certain physical signs and compiled blueprints to identify and screen them (Mosse 1990). Furthermore, it was also "deviations" in gender orientation and identity that were highlighted. "Homosexuals" and "transsexuals", who were hardly distinguished in the nineteenth century, were considered "perverted" and "degenerated" by contemporary psychiatry in the second half of the nineteenth century (Herrn 2005; Prüll 2016; Mahr and Prüll 2018).

This brings me closer to our topic: Women were the largest social group that was "different" in that it did not correspond to the common, male-connoted values in the bourgeois age of sifting, sorting and ordering. Medicine was aimed at the young man of working age. Children, women and the elderly were not given the same attention (see Jordanova 1989). Furthermore, the coupling of the organic and the spiritual components of identity also led to a typologisation, which depicted women as inferior to men. Psychiatry contributed its former knowledge. The psychiatrist Paul Möbius wrote in 1900 about the "physiological feeble-mindedness of the woman" (Möbius and de Burgos 1900). The psychiatrist

Richard von Krafft-Ebing formulated in 1890 that in women "the dangerous times of pregnancy, puerperium and climacteric assert themselves that in and of themselves the woman is physically and mentally less resistant than the man", and that furthermore, "the insanity is more inherited by the female offspring". This would, however, "be amply compensated for in the man by overexertion in the fight for existence, which he must fight through largely alone, by drunkenness, by sexual excesses, which are more offensive to the man than to the woman". If the woman alone must pass the struggle for existence, as in the case of a widow, then she succumbs more easily and more quickly than the man (von Krafft-Ebing 1890). Consequently, the social role of women was defined according to bourgeois standards, and medical measures were carried out accordingly. The male physician with his attitudes dominated all decisions concerning diagnostic and therapeutic measures for his female patients (Moscucci 1990). In a very patriarchal medicine that also experimented on patients without being asked, the latter did not have much leeway.

This changed increasingly from about 1900 in a long process. At the turn of the century, patients complained about their long stay in psychiatric institutions, and journalists wrote articles about the poor treatment of the poor in hospital. The trial of the dermatologist Albert Neisser from Wroclaw, who had experimented on underage prostitutes and was sentenced to pay a fine, marked the beginning of an increasing defensiveness of patients with regard to the defence of their rights (Elkeles 1996). Remarkably, once again it is not only a rehabilitation movement of "patients" but also of those social groups that had (and still have) a unique selling point and had (and still have) to seek special medical care.

The process of this self-empowerment took place with breaks and fluctuations and it cannot be traced in detail here. The first major peak is certainly after 1918 for the interwar period, when the Western European states and the USA pursued a "Volksfürsorge" (welfare) policy against the background of the First World War and the massive losses and privations (Peuckert 1987). In the context of this new political orientation, not only were patient rights strengthened but also those of the "othered" people. The emancipation of homosexuals, lesbians and transsexuals received an initial boost. Organisational structures were created. "Transsexuals", as they had been called since 1923, were for the first time increasingly perceived by the public and were able to receive medical help in the process of gender equality, after the way had been paved for this since the turn of the century through the work of the sexologist Magnus Hirschfeld (1868–1935) (Prüll 2016). This also applied to the situation of women, who were granted the right to vote in Germany in 1919. Above all, women took the first steps toward medical self-empowerment. In the last third of the nineteenth century, in the context of precursor developments in England and the USA, clinics were established in Berlin in which female doctors treated women. Roughly at the same time, medical studies in Germany had opened up to women, which had had been done successively in many other countries from around 1860 onwards (Hoesch 1995; Bleker 1998). In 1924, the "Deutscher Ärztebund" was founded. Also during the Weimar period, sexual counselling centres were established to support women with regard to contraception and questions about pregnancy (von Soden 1988).

The second major censorship occurred during the period after 1945, when another war had to be overcome, and as a consequence of the "German dictatorship" (Bracher 1969). This new emancipation and rehabilitation movement affected both patients and clients who had and still have to use medical services. It began as early as the 1950s, when many groups once again asserted their rights with more or less publicity. For example, when the "Deutscher Diabetikerbund" (German Diabetic Association) was founded in 1951, diabetes patients succeeded in establishing the first German patient self-help group and, above all, they were able to create their own identity by critically engaging with their therapists (Prüll 2013). The deaf, who have given themselves their own representation of interests since 1950 with the "Deutscher Gehörlosenbund e.V." are another example, illuminating that different morphological conditions are not necessarily disabilities. In the context of the disability studies they are no longer considered as "sick" but as "other" people whose rehabilitation is still ongoing (Uhlig 2012; Söderfeldt 2013).

The sequence of events mentioned above is important if one wants to understand the impact of GynePunks within the framework of the women's movement, which has just experienced a new (second) wave of the emancipation movement after the Second World War, more precisely since the 1970s. The background to this, in relation to medicine, is the feminist movement's unease with both male-dominated medical science and practice. After 1945 traditionally in standardised textbooks woman have been represented as fundamentally "different". As such they appeared as a special case that requires special treatment or attention and to study such different bodies became for young doctors a journey into the "foreign" and "mysterious" (Lupton 1995). In the field of health education and information, classic role models have been cemented (Sammer 2015; Linek and Pfütsch 2016). Therefore, the early feminist movement, within the framework of the division of "sex" and "gender", turned primarily to the latter, and thus to "the order of the genders" as a social, historically determined construct. The biological body of the woman was taken for granted in an essentialist way. It is only since the late 1970s and 1980s that this attitude has been questioned. The preoccupation with the female body exposed it as a product of time-dependent inscriptions and descriptions (Oudshoorn 2001). In this sense, feminists like Teresa de Lauretis attempt to mediate between essentialism and social constructivism by emphasising that the female body is constantly being created anew within the framework of socio-political discourses. The still male-dominated scientific system thus has no power of interpretation for the biological female body. Rather, the body is constantly being renegotiated, as are the social coordinates of gender relations (De Lauretis 1990).

This means, not least, that it has become more broadly defined what constitutes "the woman". And it also means that there is no uniform life path for women in the sense of "queerness". The bipolar gender image that was constructed in the nineteenth century is also being increasingly eroded. In this sense, GynePunk acts as a grouping that promotes the self-empowerment of women. Against the background of historical developments, this can be interpreted as a further step: While women had already sent their own actors into the medical system towards the end of the nineteenth century, it is now women without medical training who are taking possession of medicine, appropriating it, and spreading the knowledge among themselves.

Historical analyses often speak of "counter-worlds" when social groups develop their own identities and life constructions (Leonhard and Mignon Kirchhof 2015). Much more appropriate might be the term "parallel world", with which GynePunks can be placed in the various examples of "other" people presented here. Ultimately, these are negotiation processes that take place even with the controversially discussed scientific medicine. It is an attempt to establish and find acceptance in society with certain practices of the exercise of femininity. In the following section, I will examine how exactly this process took place in relation to GynePunks since the late 1960s.

4.2   Unknown Bodies

Influenced by the upheavals of the burgeoning civil rights movement, twelve women (including Jane Pincus, Ruth Davidson and Nancy Hawley) met for a workshop in Boston in 1969. This workshop had the theme "Women and their Bodies". On the fringes of the official event, which was led by Nancy Hawley, the participants shared their experiences in the health care system and with doctors (Nichols 2000; Lippman et al. 2008; Nelson 2015). They discussed the hierarchical relationship that the almost always male gynaecologists had with them, who paternalistically controlled their bodies, their health and their reproduction. The women found that this attitude of the opposite sex left them unaware of how their bodies worked and how the health care they received precisely influenced their bodies, regulated their reproductive capacity and controlled their sexual sensations (Morgen 2002). As members of an increasingly politicised middle class, they decided to change this situation. As a result of many later discussions, including at Jane Pincus' kitchen table, they agreed upon two things. First, the institutionalisation of their meetings as the Boston Women's Health Collective. Second, to conduct together a "summer experiment" (Morgen 2002). In the course of this experiment, they wanted to transform the ignorance about their own bodies into action knowledge in order to become active actors in the face of their own physicality, the health system and its paternalistically conceived form of expertise. At the beginning of the experiment, there was a more precise identification of problems and the collection of data. At the end there were practices of self-empowerment, the distribution of knowledge in self-help courses, political activism, and finally the founding of collectives in other US-American cities. In the words of the collective:

One year ago, a group of us (…) got together to work on laywoman's course on health, women and our bodies. (…) After that, several of us developed a questionnaire about women's feelings about their bodies and their relationship to doctors. We discovered there were no 'good' doctors and we had to learn for ourselves: We talked about our own experiences and we share our own knowledge. We went to books and to medically trained people for more information. We decided on the topics collectively. (Originally, they included: Patient as Victim; Sexuality; Anatomy; Birth Control; Abortion; Pregnancy; Prepared Childbirth; Postpartum and Childcare; Medical Institutions; Medical Laws; and Organising for Change) We picked the one or the ones we wanted to do and worked individually and in groups to write the papers. The process that developed in the group became as important as the material we were learning. For the first time, we were doing research and writing papers that were about us and for us. We were excited and our excitement was powerful. We wanted to share both the excitement and the material we were learning with our sisters. We saw ourselves differently and our lives began to change. As we worked, we met weekly to discuss what we were learning about ourselves, our bodies, health and women. We presented each topic to the group, gave support and helpful criticisms to each other and rewrote the papers. By the fall, we were ready to share our collective knowledge with our sisters. Excited and nervous (we were just women; what authority did we have in matters of medicine and health?), we offered a course to sisters in women's liberation. Singularly and in groups, we presented the topics and discussed the material; sometimes in one large group, often in smaller groups. Sisters added their experiences, questions, fears, feelings, excitement. It was dynamic! We all learned together. One original version (sic!) of the course was that we as a group would give the course to a group of women who could then go out and give it to other women. (Boston Women's Health Collective 1970: 3)

The self-help course described in the quote, one of the first of its kind, and the accompanying practices of knowledge search, knowledge discussion, and knowledge distribution are key elements in understanding the activism of the early Women's Health Movement. The women involved were not only active in learning more about themselves and their own bodies, but also decided early on that what they had learned should be shared with other women to give them the opportunity to learn more about their own bodies, independent of medical expertise. The revolutionary act was that they began to produce collective knowledge for a marginalised population, of which they themselves were a part, by not only acquiring and sharing discursive knowledge but also testing it on the very practical level of their own needs. They did not stop at the use and reinterpretation of esoteric medical practices, which were kept in a kind of black box by the medical system. For this purpose they developed simple but effective practices of self-empowerment.

For Carol Downer, a working-class housewife who had previously worked as a women's rights activist at the discourse level, the process of the shared acquisition of medical knowledge through simple practices was a moment of awakening. In Sandra Morgen's book Into Our Own Hands (2002), she relates that she was a guest in a friend's kitchen and participated with some other women from the neighbourhood in the first cervix self-examination of her neighbourhood. She describes what she experienced when one of her neighbours examined herself and felt as follows:

> There she was up in the stirrups, with a speculum in, and there, voila, was a cervix. I think the reason it had such a momentous impact on me is that I was going out and doing all this public speaking and looking at it (the need for abortion) so intellectually, so politically. And then to see how beautiful and simple and accessible a cervix was overwhelmed me with the significance of it (…) I immediately ran out and told every women friend I had, this is going to change everything. (Downer 1990, quoted after Morgen 2002)

Downer, who had been pregnant several times in her life, had never seen a cervix in her life. This privilege had previously only been granted to her gynaecologists, who used their stainless steel instruments, shielded by a white cloth, to explore, examine and evaluate the de-individualised body in front of them (Morgen 2002). In her book "Vaginal Politics", author Ellen Frankfort illustrates the contrast between the two settings very clearly:

It was a little like having a blind person see for the first time – for what woman is not blind to her own insides? The simplicity (…) brought forth in a flash the whole gynecological ritual: the receptionist, the magazines, the waiting room, and then the examination itself – being told to undress, lying on your back with your feet in the stirrups, looking at a blank ceiling while waiting in an overly air-conditioned room (the doctor isn't the one without clothes, after all) for him to enter – and no one thinking that 'meeting' a doctor for the first time in this position is slightly odd. (…) (N) ot only does the drapery further depersonalise the woman by making her faceless and bodiless except for her vagina, it also prevents her from seeing what the doctor is doing. (Frankfort 1972)

Given her experience in her friend's kitchen, Downer quickly understood how easy it would be to take her reproductive life into her own hands. Easy-to-learn knowledge and a little technology, such as the use of a speculum, a simple hand mirror, and a standard flashlight, were all that was needed (Morgen 2002). This practical knowledge quickly made the rounds, not only in Downer's neighbourhood but also in other places. Women all over the country began to explore their cervix and other organs of their reproductive system in small groups (initially under the guidance of multipliers) and to acquire the necessary know-how for their own health care. Examples of this know how include the early detection of inflammations or fungal infections. In the process of studying their own bodies regularly, they finally developed their own "standpoint expertise".

In this learning and examination context, the women also jointly developed strategies for civil disobedience to the health care system. Although these strategies were initially low-threshold, but they were quite effective on the individual level of self-awareness, as they played with both medical expectations and the health care system, which was structured by state. According to Frankfort, Downer and her colleagues advised the women to behave as follows when they needed to visit a gynaecologist

Carol and Lorraine advise women to discard the drape by throwing it on the floor when the doctor enters. If he replaces it, throw it on the floor again. If he questions your behaviour, tell him that doctors in California are no longer draping. And if you're in California, tell him that doctors in New York have stopped this strange custom. (Frankfort 1972)

In 1973, twelve hundred women's health groups had already been founded in the USA (Baxandall and Gordon 2020). Groups such as the Boston Women's Health Collective travelled around and procured cheap plastic specula for the women who came to their seminars (Frankfort 1972). These had become an easily accessible and affordable mass product by the time of the US Patent 3745992 A (filed by J. Poirier) and the mass distribution by Medical Specialities Inc. in 1971. This represented a remarkable overlap between the mass availability of a technology and the possibility of technology-induced participation through its appropriation. Interestingly, we are experiencing similar phenomena again today, at least on the discursive level (Bass et al. 2013; Kullenberg and Kasperowsky 2016). The New York Times journalist and feminist author Ellen Frankfort describes in her 1973 article Medicine, the Feminist Frontier how the activist knowledge practice of female self-empowerment by means of the speculum actually looked and what changed it. She illustrates the social situations in which it occurred:

Recently, small teams of women have been traveling across the country equipped with a plastic speculum, mirrors and flashlight. In informal settings, surrounded by the curious, they show how a woman can observe her own cervix. I hesitate to use the word 'revolutionary' but no other seems accurate to describe the effects of the demonstration. It is, in fact, a little like having a blind person see for the first time – for what woman is not blind to her own insides? Since the first demonstration two years ago, the interest in 'self-help' (as it's comes to be known) has spread throughout the country (…). (Frankfort 1973)

Under the heading of self-help, light was thrown into the black box of the female body by those who actually "lived" these bodies, but to whom it was previously only accessible (if at all) in a physician-dominated and reductionist perspective. At the same time, Frankfort refers to the spread, radiance and ultimately also to the beginning institutionalisation of the movement. In the following section of her article, she finally presents contextualising considerations on how medical expertise is deconstructed and reconfigured through the self-help practices of women's collectives, with social and also epistemological consequences. Frankfort understands the performative-paternalistic exclusion of women as active actors in the health care system from a social perspective as a further episode in the struggle for equality and educational opportunities led in the early 1970s. The aim is to bring about a change in the system, which still focuses on illness rather than prevention, by leaving people in the dark about their own bodies and allowing only highly specialised people to examine their bodies. According to Frankfort, the demystification of medicine is an essential task of the civil rights and equality movement, which must also be structurally linked to educational strategies and educational opportunities for women (Frankfort 1973).

For Frankfort, however, the female perspective on her own body also has potential in epistemic terms is that it has enabled the discovery of new phenomena and practices that would not be possible without the specifically lived experiences and questions about her own physicality. For example, the practice of reducing menstruation by extraction. Such discovery of new practices and alternative knowledge has become one of the main arguments for integrating the "diversity of perspectives" as an epistemic value into the production of scientific and medical knowledge, as feminist theory would also demand a few years later (Longino 1990, 1994, 1995; Hekman 1997). Frankfort writes:

> Along with self-examination, the self-help women have pioneered a new technique of great interest: menstrual extraction. For two years, several women have been reducing their menstrual flow to half an hour by aspirating out the lining of the uterus. (Frankfort 1973)

However, as a critical activist and feminist, whose work vehemently advocates the sustainable integration of feminist voices in health policy (Frankfort 1972), Frankfort also recognises problems in the practices of female self-help groups, which often rely solely on the experience of relatively small groups. She therefore calls for this knowledge to be integrated into a broader scientific, political and socially sensitive context, albeit in a decidedly feminist way. If self-help were to remain in living rooms, kitchens, and basements, the larger goal of improving the health of women at all levels would ultimately be jeopardised:

> Yet it is still impossible to find out even the most simple fact: How regularly? Are there any hormonal changes noted? What is done when complications arise? How would women react if a group of men came by with a technique they had been practicing for two years, and, with almost no additional information beyond what they personally experienced, recommended that we experiment with it on ourselves or with one another.
>
> Feminist politics cannot be divorced from other political realities. Doctors, hospitals and drug companies are not going to be affected by having small groups of women learning to examine themselves or how to extract their menstrual periods. Nor will such self-help improve health care for the people who lack the kind of movement experience that leads to feeling at ease with women working in homes without supervision. And it will not help the women (and men) who are too sick for self-help and who have no alternative but to go to a hospital. In order to receive the best care, people must receive not only dignified, non-patronising, nonsexist care but also medically sound care that takes into account the latest scientific knowledge. (Frankfort 1973)

Demands like these set two processes in motion within the self-help scene. What both have in common is that they heralded a new phase of the Women's Health Movement and each produced a new type of activist. First, there was an increased politicisation of the movement by political women's health activists who wanted to bring "women's issues" into the medical, scientific and political system and to change "the system from within" (Verbrugge 1982; Mulligan 1983; Ehrenreich 1984; Seaman 1995 [1975]).

Another way was the institutionalisation of self-help parallel to the established medical system. However, it was to remain in the hands of independent women. This path was advocated for and pursued by those activists who worried that the medical system was not yet ready for reforms from within. These women were responsible for the founding of the so-called Feminist Health Clinics, which were especially dedicated to the need for protection of women from marginalised social groups and women in difficult life situations. In other words, such clinics catered to people who do not have access to classical medical institutions or who might perceive them as alienating and hostile. Consequently, the clinics were planned as a counter-draft to the state medical system at the institutional level (Marieskind and Ehrenreich 1975; Span 1980). In the July 1973 issue of Sister magazine, published by the Los Angeles Women's Center, the goals of the clinics were as follows. It is now considered an expression of the militant spirit of self-help:

> The goal of the Self-Help Clinic (is) to take women's medicine back into our own hands The strategy is to take back the power over our own bodies, both everyday types of control which information and self-knowledge gives us, and we also want to acquire special skills and knowledge which will allow us collectively to independently provide our health care. To implement this strategy we have given Self-Help Clinic presentations, started Self-Help Clinics, set up abortion referral services and abortion clinics, given childbirth conferences, and established health centres as bases of operations. None of these activities are ends in themselves. In contrast to some women's action groups who have formed to 'start a clinic' or to 'write a book', we develop tactics to further the struggle. We are a spearhead of social change.
>
> The spirit of Self-Help is aggressive and positive. We believe that it is good for women to be powerful. It is not only our basic right to have good health, recreation, knowledge, communication, pleasure – it is absolutely essential that we have all these good 'inputs' to make a vigorous and successful effort to get social change. (Los Angeles Women's Center 1973)

4.3   Feminist Symbolism

If one follows the remarks of historian Jill Lepore in her book The Secret History of Wonder Woman (2015), two things in particular became iconic for the fierce and positive character of self-help. The first was the superhero character Wonder Women, as an equally feminine, emancipated but also powerful woman. The second was the speculum, a tool that has initially been a symbol for the dominance of male access to female bodies and female health but which recently had undergone the transformation into a symbol of female sisterhood, ingenuity, and bodily empowerment. Due to due to its simple usability, availability and distribution in plastic it was charged with the hope that women could finally become the knowledgeable mistresses of their own physicality. This is impressively illustrated on the cover of the June (1973) issue of the magazine Sister (Fig. 4.1).

Here we encounter the comic figure Wonder Women in her typical ambivalent robes, a mixture of feminised breastplate, a tiara and high-heeled boots, all patterned in the style of the star banner. A woman who at the same time appears strong, sexy, self-determined and, due to the

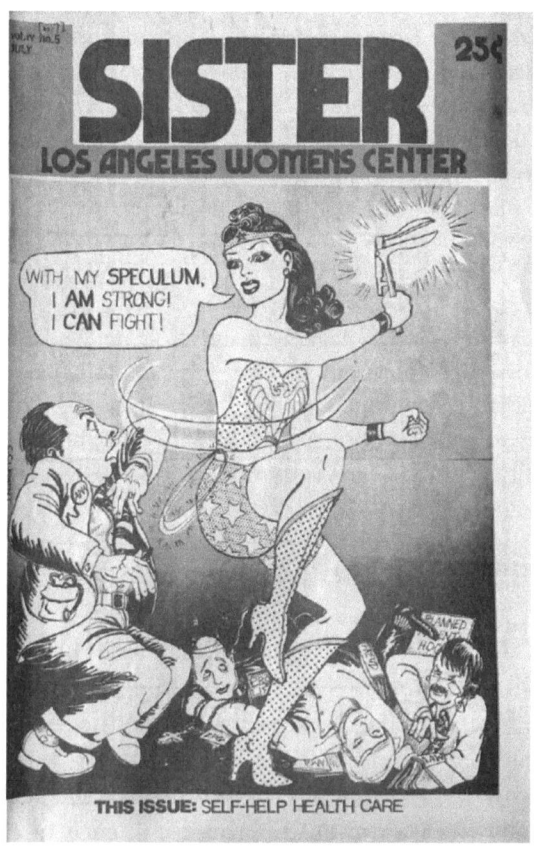

Fig. 4.1 Cover of the July 1973 issue of Sister magazine. (Los Angeles Women's Center 1973)

spirit of the times, patriotic, thus questioning already classic gender roles. This was also intended by the creator of her figure, the psychologist Wiliam Moulton Marston (1893–1947) (Lepore 2015). One thing, however, is slightly altered in this iconography typical of her. For, instead of her actual weapon, the "Lasso of Truth", she carries a radiant speculum and uses it to fight some shady characters. Some of these figures lie on the ground, struck down by the warrior, who is shown enlarged in terms of perspective and positioned centrally in the picture. She shouts: "With my Speculum, I am Strong! I can Fight!" (Los Angeles Women's Center 1973). A closer look at her opponents reveals that they are representatives of the political, medical and cultural system of the USA in the 1970s. This is made clear to the viewers of the cover through insignia, references, key words and abbreviations. Already on the ground are a bespectacled psychologist with a "Freud" book at his side, a blond man in a kind of white uniform surrounded by books as well as brochures with the titles "Law", "AMA", "ZPG" (Zero Population Growth), "Planned Parenthood", and a Catholic priest with a rosary and a book entitled "Pro Live". Still in battle, the warrior princess is struggling with a bald gentleman who has a stethoscope in his suit pocket and a button with "AMA" written on his lapel.

Wonder Women appears in the picture as a dialectical figure. She is simultaneously a symbol of the Women's Health Movement with its past successes (since 1969) and a figure of identification for each individual viewer. The fight against the American Medical Association (AMA) has already been won in parts (brochure on the floor) but is continuing (the still standing opponent). Whereas the opponents of abortion are already on the ground. The same applies to psychotherapy and psychiatry, which at that time still operated with concepts such as "female hysteria" but were actively and conceptually challenged by the Feminist Counselling Collectives within the Women's Health Movement (The Feminist Counselling Collective 1975). The fact that Wonder Women's struggle against the "AMA" is not yet completely over sends out a signal that the movement is still looking for allies. But one doesn't become an ally only through political activism but rather the "fight" still endures through the acquisition of self-knowledge. For this, the speculum and its history is a symbol in its own right. It is no coincidence that the speculum shines in the cover illustration with an "aureole", as it was used in art history for depictions of saints and Christ himself. It reveals, as it were, masculine forms of expertise and the oppressive potentials in the medical system associated with them.

Women's Health Movement Reloaded?

Let us leave the 1970s for a moment and take a leap into our own decade. Here we will examine whether the GynePunks mentioned in the introduction embody a similar form of activism as the Women's Health Movement. Let us first take a look at the self-portrayal of the Spanish health activists. On their homepage calafou.org the group defines the term GynePunk:

> GynePunk is about engaging in a radical change of perspective about medical technologies, and the so-called 'professional' and medical institutions. GynePunk is an extreme and accurate gesture to detach our bodies from the compulsive dependency of the fossil structures of the hegemonic health system machine. GynePunk's objective is to enable the emergence of DIY-DIT accessible diagnosis labs and techniques in extreme experimentation spaces, down on the rocks or in elevators if it is necessary. It is about having these possibilities in a situated stable place or/and in nomadic mobile labs to be able to perform as much as WE WANT, in an intensive way: smears, fluid analysis, biopsy, PAPs, synthesise hormones at will, blood tests, urinalysis, HIV tests, pain relief, or whatever WE NEED. It is about hacking and building our own ultrasound, endoscope or echography devices in a low-cost way. All this experimentation is made in complementarity with herbs and natural knowledges, oral traditions, underground recipes, seeking with hunger to generate a plethora of DIY lubricants, anti-contraceptives, open doula domains, savage caring of any visceral hands-on technologies, such as menstrual extraction, all elevated to the maximum potential of common learning and radical self-body-power ...! (Colonia ecoindustrial postcapitalista 2014)

The GynePunks, like Carol Downer and the collectives of the 1970s, are thus concerned with taking their bodily agency back into their own hands and thus taking action against a system of expertise and epistemic institutions that they perceive as oppressive and paternalistic. Like their predecessors, they mark the appropriation of technology as an essential tool for this, even if the catalogue of these tools (DIY ultrasound devices, centrifuges, etc.) is drastically expanded in comparison to those of the past (hand mirrors from the drugstore, kitchen utensils and specula from the mail-order business). In addition, one's own actions are placed in the contemporary context of the hacker ethos and the eco-economic secondary use of technological artefacts (Delfanti 2013). Consequently, today's activism no longer takes place in the home kitchen or a self-help clinic, but in a garage or a biohacking laboratory. The search for self-determined spaces of health participation is nevertheless functionally equivalent in both temporal horizons.

The same seems to be true for the dependence on specific techno-cultural conditions; in the 1970s, it was the easy availability of plastic specula, in the present, an almost limitless availability of open source building instructions for the creative misuse of technical artefacts. In the hands of activists, these become centrifuges and other medical devices (Fig. 4.2). Not only the acquisition and application of medical knowledge but also the know-how for the construction of technical equipment is important for the TransHackFeminism. This is accompanied by a subtle but significant difference in the social structure of activism, which influences its goals and reach. Even though we are surrounded by a multitude of technical artefacts every day, very few of us are able to easily misuse a technical artefacts in a creative way, no matter how accessible the building instructions are.

The creative-avant-garde moment of the hacker ethos thus limits the reach of activism. This in turn means that the GynePunks live predominantly for themselves or are at most active as agents for their target groups, whereas the early Women's Health Movement was (at least in part) "the concerned people themselves". This is because the material that was used at that time for physical self-empowerment could be directly used. Knowing how to make your own tools was not mandatory. This is an important difference that I will discuss in more detail below. But first I would like to dwell a little on the similarities between the two

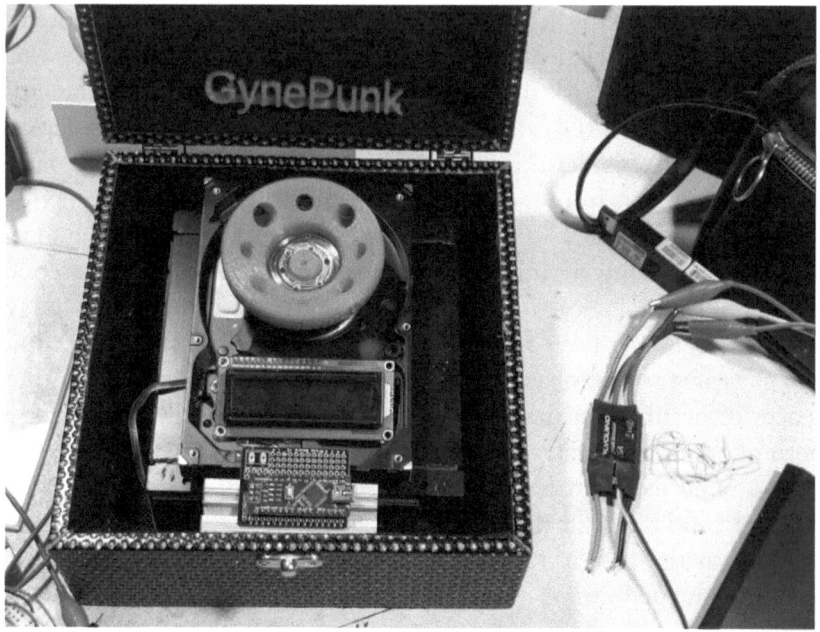

Fig. 4.2 Hard disk motor converted to a centrifuge with a sample holder from the 3D. (Photo: Paula Pin/Creative Commons License)

movements. These lie both in the performative and in the respective iconography and symbolism.

The performative element of both movements knows two interwoven main levels: seminars, which are intended to impart basic medical knowledge, and the partially public exploration of female physicality that takes place within this framework. This serves both as an act of self-empowerment and as an opportunity for independent health care. In addition, there is an outwardly directed photographic documentation of these acts, which, on the one hand, is intended to clarify the majority society's own claims, but on the other hand also addresses women (and in the case of GynePunks other vulnerable groups) as potential participants/activists. In the two figures below (4.3 and 4.4) we see how GynePunks carry out the examination of their own bodies. In Figs. 4.5 and 4.6 we find for comparison two photos of self-examination of women in the

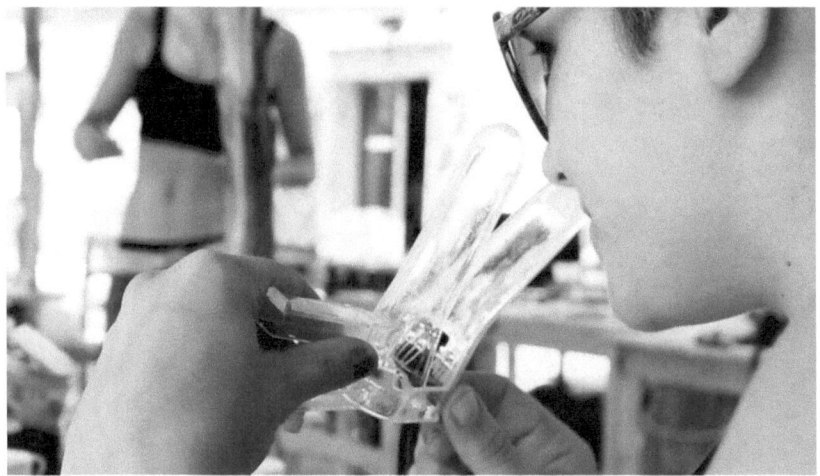

Fig. 4.3 TransHackAktivist_in (2014) installing a webcam in a plastic speculum shortly before performing a Vinegar test on another activist. (Photo: Paula Pin/ Creative Commons License)

1970s. The similarities are obvious. However, there are also remarkable differences.

The similarity of the performative act is astonishing in both cases. Female physicality is openly represented. Nudity and examination are not de-individualised, but are presented and documented in an unembellished way. In both time contexts, the speculum functions as a connecting symbol. However, in each case something additional is transported. In the representations of the GynePunks, one can observe a certain technophilia and countercultural performance. In contrast, we observe an educational seriousness in the photos form the 1970s. These noticeable divergences underscore the expression of two different forms of the demand for participation in the health care system, each of which is dependent on time and context. On the one hand, participation as a highly individualised performative act of breaking out in the context of a medicine whose suppressive potential lies in the implicit demands for self-observation and self-regulation (twenty-first century) (Dubriwny 2013); on the other hand, participation as understood as participation of

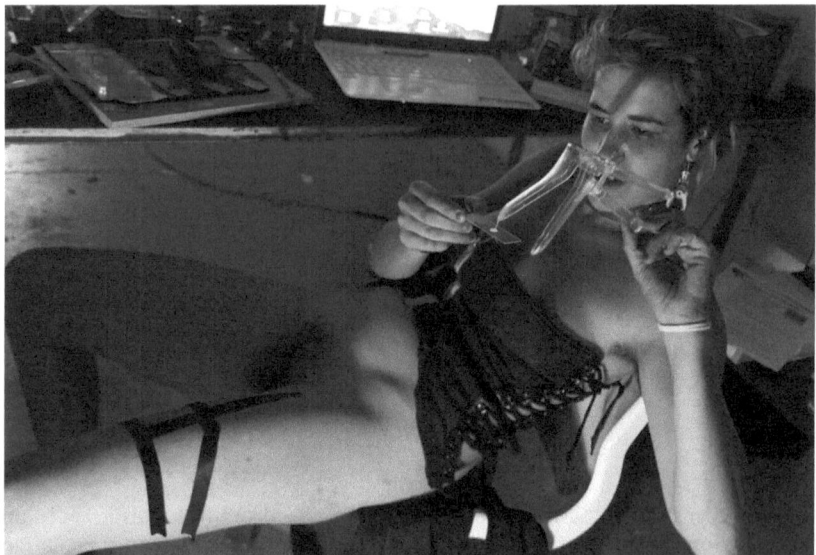

Fig. 4.4 Swab using a plastic speculum in Ca la Fou (2014). (Photo: Paula Pin/ Creative Commons License)

one's own structurally marginalised group in the health care system (Morgen 2002).

The difference between performativity and education, can further be illustrated by the GynePunks' affinity for technology. It is precisely this characteristic that limits the range of participation that they make possible. Although the activists from Calafou want to develop cheap technologies for marginalised groups such as sex workers, migrants, and so forth, these target groups do not always have access to elaborate technical knowhow or equipment such as 3D printers. Therefore, the GynePunks remain, at least for now, a rather avant-garde group in terms of their forms of expression and influence. This group provides technologies and knowledge, but they are not easily operationalised by everyone. Participation is rather realised against the background of the possibilities of an origin from the context of the "bohemian bourgeois". An example of this can be seen in the DIY centrifuge displayed in figure number 4.2.

The speculum, on the other hand, is what really makes participation equally possible in both time frames. It is no coincidence that the

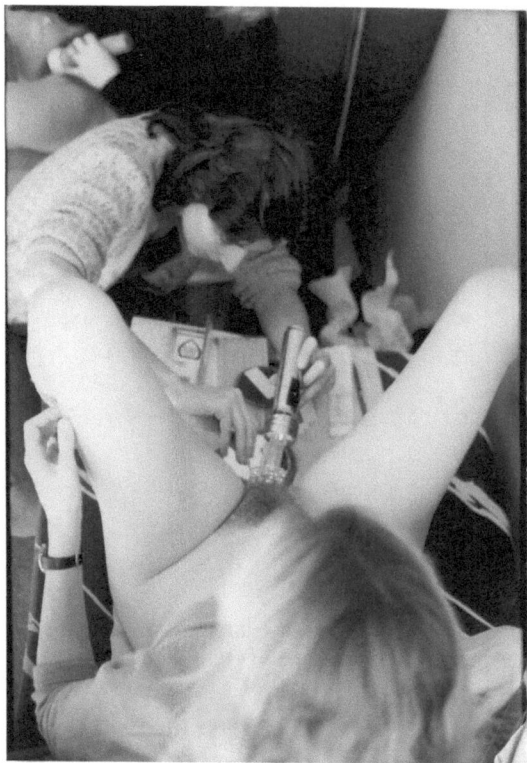

Fig. 4.5   Self-examination using a plastic speculum and a flashlight (1971). (Photo: www.womwenshealthinwomenshands.org (2011))

speculum is a central iconographic element in many depictions. In the case of the GynePunks it is sometimes also upgraded as a DIY object and is made simultaneously steadily available (as an idea and print instructions) and yet paradoxically unavailable (dependence on access to 3D printers) (see Fig. 4.7).

Nevertheless, it conveys feminist claims to participation in one's own physicality and in the health care system. For example, it appears not only on the cover of the 1973 magazine "Sister" but also as a design element of the event poster for the TransHackFeminist Convergence in 2014 (Fig. 4.8).

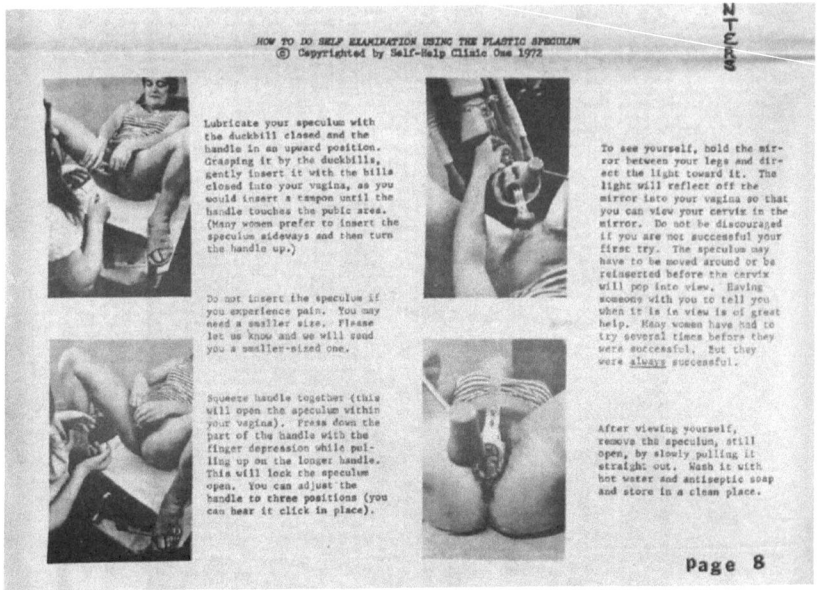

Fig. 4.6 Illustrated instructions for self-examination using a speculum published in: "Sister" July issue 1973. (Copyright Self-Help Clinic One 1972)

4.4 Conclusion

Does TransHackFeminism thus enable a completely new form of participation in one's own physicality on the one hand and the health system on the other? This question cannot be answered in the affirmative without reservation. It could be shown that the GynePunks stand in a historical tradition in which they ask and answer classical questions about women's access to their own bodies. The programmatic objective of self-empowerment is thus old, and the motive of reconquering one's own body as resistance to a health system perceived as oppressive is also not new. The Women's Health Movement of the 1960s and 1970s was already committed to this goal. However, GynePunk is an avant-garde movement, which claims that the body should be examined by female laypeople. This perspective is new, even though the symbolism (the speculum) is very similar to that of the old women's health movement, and the rhetoric is analogous.

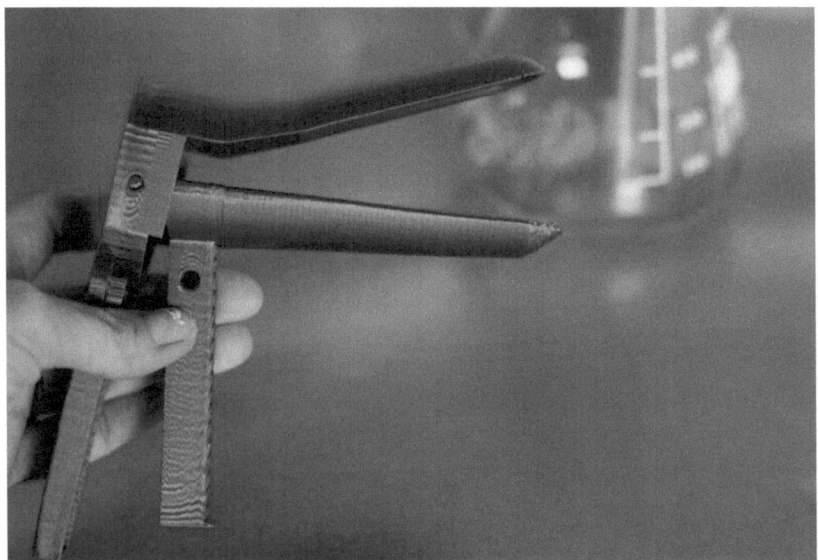

Fig. 4.7 Speculum from the 3D printer (Design: GaudiLabs). (Photo: Klau Kinky/ Creative Commons License)

Why are these practices so relevant today? Haven't our (Western) health care systems become more open and multi-perspective since the 1970s, when Carol Downer, Jane Pincus, Nancy Hawley and ultimately many thousands of other women struggled for recognition of their own physicality? Not quite. The reality is that our multidimensional medicine of the present is ambivalent. On the one hand, it complies with what the activists of the 1970s demanded, that is it focuses on prevention, it is predictive and to a certain extent has recently become participatory. But at the same time, these qualities have become part of an unconstrained compulsion towards self-regulation, which has a similarly oppressive effect on women's health and the health of and minority groups health as the epistemic paternalism of the past.

As a symbolic-paradoxical intervention, the GynePunks with their uneasiness against the system thus come at the right time. However, they remain self-referential through their own affinity for technology. Certainly, one problem here is that the unlimited availability of open source manuals and blueprints for 3D printers is not true for many

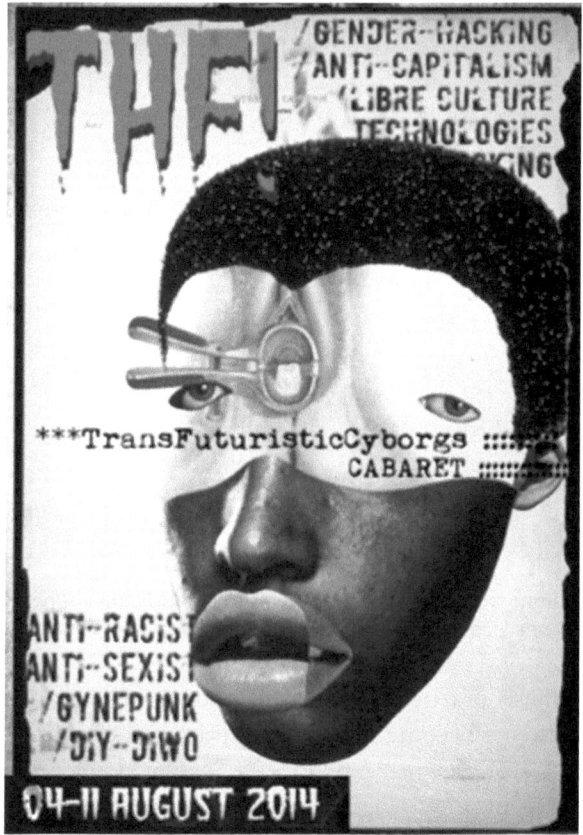

Fig. 4.8 Event poster of the GynePunk Movement (2014). (Source: https://cala-fou.org/)

individuals within the very marginalised demographics they target with their activism. The activism of alternative social health movements, such as the GynePunks, should realise that "openness technology" in the western sense does not necessarily translate into other cultural and social contexts. For this, it is important to find local solutions by the local populations for the local populations. An example of this is the Thai Baan research, which I will describe in more detail in the following chapter.

References

Bass, Emily, Burns Julien, and Deidre Grant. 2013. Citizen Scientists and Activist Researchers: Building and Sustaining HIV Prevention Research Advocacy in the Era of Evidence. In *Global HIV/AIDS Politics, Policy, and Activism, 3: Activism and Community Mobilization*, ed. A. Raymond, 135–156. Santa Barbara: Praeger.

Baxandall, Rosalyn, and Linda Gordon. 2020. *Dear Sisters. Dispatches form the Women's Liberation Movement*. New York: Basic Books.

Bierend, Dough. 2015. Meet the GynePunks Pushing the Boundaries of DIY Gynecology. *Motherboard* (online). http://motherboard.vice.com/read/meet-the-gynepunks-pushing-the-boundaries-of-diy-gynecology. Accessed 18 Dec 2020.

Bleker, Johanna. 1998. *Der Eintritt der Frauen in die Gelehrtenrepublik. Zur Geschlechterfrage im akademischen Selbstverständnis und in der wissenschaftlichen Praxis am Anfang des 20. Jahrhunderts*. Abhandlungen zur Geschichte der Medizin und der Naturwissenschaften 84. Husum: Matthiesen.

Boston Women's Health Collective. 1970. *Women and Their Bodies: A Course*. Boston: BWHC.

Bracher, Karl-Dietrich. 1969. *Die deutsche Diktatur: Entstehung, Struktur, Folgen des Nationalsozialismus*. Köln: Kieenheuer & Witsch.

Bynum, William F. 1994. *Science and the Practice of Medicine in the Nineteenth Century*. Cambridge: Cambridge University Press.

Bynum, William F., Anne Hardy, Stephen Jacyna, Christopher Lawrence, and E.M. Tilli. 2006. *The Western Medical Tradition. 1800 to 2000*. Cambridge: Cambridge University Press.

Colonia ecoindustrial postcapitalista. 2014. *A TransHackFeminist (THF!) Convergence Report from Calafou*. https://calafou.org/en/content/transhackfeminist-thf-convergence-report. Accessed 9 Dec 2020.

De Lauretis, Teresa. 1990. Upping the Anti in Feminist Theory. In *Conflicts in Feminism*, ed. Marianne Hirsch and Evelyn Fox Keller, 255–270. London: Routledge.

Delfanti, Alessandro. 2013. *Biohackers. The Politics of Open Science*. London: Pluto Press.

Dubriwny, Tasha N. 2013. *The Vulnerable Empowered Woman: Feminism, Postfeminism, and Women's Health*, Critical Issues in Health and Medicine. New Brunswick: Rutgers University Press.

Ehrenreich, Barbara. 1984. Body Politic: The Growth of the Women's Health Movement. *Ms. Magazine.* http://www.msmagazine.com/spring2002/ehrenreichandfuntes.asp. Accessed 9 Dec 2020.

Elkeles, Barbara. 1996. *Der moralische Diskurs über das medizinische Menschenexperiment im 19. Jahrhundert.* Stuttgart: Fischer.

Frankfort, Ellen. 1972. *Vaginal Politics. Who Controls a Woman's Body: Doctors? Lovers? Drugs? Women?* New York: Bantam Books.

———. 1973. Medicine, the Feminist Frontier. *The New York Times*, March 3.

Hekman, Susan. 1997. Truth and Method: Feminist Standpoint Theory Revisited. *Signs* 22 (2): 341–365.

Herrn, Rainer. 2005. *Schnittmuster des Geschlechts. Transvestitismus und Transsexualität in der frühen Sexualwissenschaft.* Gießen: Psychosozial-Verlag.

Hoesch, Kristin. 1995. *Ärztinnen für Frauen. Kliniken in Berlin 1877–1914.* Stuttgart/Weimar: Metzler.

Jen, Clare. 2015. Do-It-Yourself Biology, Garage Biology, and Kitchen Science – A Feminist Analysis of Bio-Making Narratives. In *Knowing New Biotechnologies: Social Aspects of Technological Convergence, Genetics and Society,* ed. Matthias Wienroth and Eugenia Rorigues, 125–141. London/New York: Routledge/Taylor & Francis Group.

Jordanova, Ludmilla. 1989. *Sexual Visions. Images of Gender in Science and Medicine Between the Eighteenth and Twentieth Centuries.* Madison: University of Wisconsin Press.

Kullenberg, Christopher, and Dick Kasperowski. 2016. What Is Citizen Science? – A Scientometric Meta-Analysis. *PLoS One* 11 (1): e0147152. https://doi.org/10.1371/journal.pone.0147152. Accessed 18 Dec 2020.

Labisch, Alfons. 1991. Der öffentliche Gesundheitsdienst (öGD) angesichts neuer öffentlicher Gesundheitsleistungen ("new public health"). In *Oeffentliche Gesundheit - Public Health - Konzepte und Diskussionen in der deutschen Geschichte*, 84–102. Frankfurt a. M.: Campus.

Leonhard, Nina, and Astrid Mignon Kirchhof. 2015. Einführung: Gegenwelten. *Geschichte und Gesellschaft* 41: 5–16.

Lepore, Jill. 2015. *The Secret History of Wonder Woman.* First Vintage Books ed. New York: Vintage Books, A Division of Random House LLC.

Lewis, Tania. 2006. DIY Selves? Reflexivity and Habitus in Young People's Use of the Internet for Health Information. *European Journal of Cultural Studies* 9 (4): 461–479.

Linek, Jenny, and Pierre Pfütsch. 2016. Geschlechterbilder in der Gesundheitsaufklärung im deutsch-deutschen Vergleich (1949–1990). *Medizin, Gesellschaft und Geschichte* 34: 73–110.

Lippman, Abby, Anne Rochon Ford, and Kathleen O'Grady. 2008. Barbara Seaman (1935–2008): Pioneer in the Women's Health Movement. *Network Magazine of the Canadian Women's Health Network* 10 (2): 18–19.

Longino, Helen. 1990. *Science as Social Knowledge: Values and Objectivity in Scientific Inquiry*. Princeton: Princeton University Press.

———. 1994. In Search of Feminist Epistemology. *The Monist* 77 (4): 472–458.

———. 1995. Gender, Politics, and the Theoretical Virtues. *Synthese* 104 (3): 383–397.

Los Angeles Womens Center. 1973. *Sister: Self-Help Health Care 4*. Los Angeles.

Lupton, Deborah. 1995. *Medicine as Culture. Illness, Disease and the Body in Western Societies*. London/Thousand Oaks/New Delhi: Sage.

Mahr, Dana, and Livia Prüll. 2018. Körperliche Selbstermächtigung aus dem 3D-Drucker? Feministische Kulturen als Parallelwelten und der Kampf um gesellschaftliche Teilhabe seit 1970. In *Kybernetik, Kapitalismus, Revolutionen. Emanzipatorische Perspektiven im technologischen Wandel*, ed. Paul Buckermann, Anne Koppenburg, and Simon Schaub, 161–190. Münster: Unrast.

Marieskind, Helen I., and Barbara Ehrenreich. 1975. Toward Socialist Medicine: The Women's Health Movement. *Social Policy* 6 (2): 34–42.

Möbius, Paul Julius, and Carmen de Burgos. 1900. *La inferioridad mental la mujer: (la deficiencia mental fisiologica de la mujer)*. F. Sempere y Cia.

Morgen, Sandra. 2002. *Into Our Own Hands: The Women's Health Movement in the United States, 1969–1990*. New Brunswick: Rutgers University Press.

Moscucci, Ornella. 1990. *The Science of Women: Gynaecology and Gender in England, 1800–1929*. Cambridge: Cambridge University Press.

Mosse, George L. 1990. *Die Geschichte des Rassismus in Europa*. Frankfurt a. M.: Suhrkamp.

Mulligan, Lesa Jean. 1983. Some Effects of the Women's Health Movement. *Topics in Clinical Nursing* 4 (4): 1–9.

Nelson, Jennifer. 2015. *More than Medicine: A History of the Feminist Women's Health Movement*. New York: New York University Press.

Nichols, Francis H. 2000. History of the Women's Health Movement in the 20th Century. *Journal of Obstetric, Gynecologic, and Neonatal Nursing* 29 (1): 56–64.

Oudshoorn, Nelly. 2001. On Bodies, Technology and Feminism. In *Feminism in Twentieth Century Science, Technology and Medicine*, ed. Angela N.H. Creager, Elizabeth Lunbeck, and Londa Schiebinger, 199–213. Chicago/London: University of Chicago Press.

Peuckert, Detlev. 1987. *Die Weimarer Republik: Krisenjahre der Klassischen Moderne*. Frankfurt a. M.: Suhrkamp.

Planert, Ute. 2000. Der dreifache Körper des Volkes: Sexualität, Biopolitik und die Wissenschaften vom Leben. *Geschichte und Gesellschaft* 26: 539–576.

Prüll, Livia. 2016. *Trans* im Glück. Geschlechtsangleichung als Chance. Autobiographie, Medizingeschichte, Medizinethik*. Göttingen: Vandenhoeck & Ruprecht.

Prüll, Cay-Rüdiger (now Livia Prüll). 2013. Making Sense of Diabetes: Public Discussions in early West Germany 1945 to 1970. In *Making Sense as a Cultural Practice*, ed. Jörg Rogge, 225–239. Bielefeld: Transcript.

Sammer, Christian. 2015. Die "Modernisierung" der Gesundheitsaufklärung in beiden deutschen Staaten zwischen 1949 und 1975. *Medizinhistorisches Journal* 50: 249–294.

Seaman, Barbara. 1995 (=1975). *The Doctor's Case Against the Pill*. 25th anniversary ed. Alameda and Emeryville Hunter House, Publishers Group West.

Söderfeldt, Ylva. 2013. *From Pathology to Public Sphere. The German Deaf Movement 1848–1914*. Bielefeld: Transcript.

Span, Paula. 1980. A New Era for Feminist Health Clinics. *The New York Times*, November 23.

The Feminist Counselling Collective. 1975. Feminist Psychotherapy. *Social Policy* 6 (2): 54–62.

Uhlig, Anne C. 2012. *Ethnographie der Gehörlosen. Kultur – Kommunikation – Gemeinschaft*. Bielefeld: Transcript.

Verbrugge, Lois M. 1982. The Women's Health Movement: Feminist Alternatives to Medical Control. *Sex Roles* 8 (2): 222–224.

von Krafft-Ebing, Richard. 1890. *Lehrbuch der Psychiatrie. Auf klinischer Grundlage für praktische Ärzte und Studierende*. 4th ed. Stuttgart: Enke.

von Soden, Kristine. 1988. *Die Sexualberatungsstellen der Weimarer Republik 1919–1933*. Berlin: Edition Hentrich.

Wohlsen, Marcus. 2011. Biopunk Kitchen-Counter Scientists Hack the Software of Life. *New York: Current* (online). https://www.overdrive.com/search?q=ACF7EAFA-86D0-402C-BB5A-EDAD02D44D4C. Accessed 18 Dec 2020.

5

Thai Baan Research: Locality as a Key for Diversity

Abstract The aim of this chapter is to investigate forms of scientific knowledge production that are only minimally influenced by western influences. An example of this is the radically localised Thai Baan research in the Mekong Delta which maps and monitors the complex ecological network of the Mekong Delta without the influence of Western scientists. Hereby they seek to improve their own living conditions on their own terms. This form of villager research differs from western democratisation programs, such as citizen science, in that it is organised entirely bottom-up on the one hand and sees itself as political activism. A prevailing question of this chapter and throughout the book will be the interrogation of what Western science can learn from this kind of non-Western approach and research. The case studies in this chapter will also be based on interviews and archival research.

Keywords Non-western epistemology • Ecology • Public participation • Villager research

It is not only in the "Global North" that new ways of doing science are being developed. Although the epistemic elements of imperialism still persists in many societies of the "Global South" today, alternative forms of knowledge have never completely disappeared there. Popular examples of this tenacity of existence are the survival of traditional medicine in China or Ayurveda in large parts of India (Stollberg 2001). However, even outside of medical practice, more and more people in these cultures begin to recall lost epistemic traditions that are independent of (and/or complementary to) European and American influences. Paradigmatic for this is the project "Ngan Wijai Thai Baan" (งานวิจัยไทบ้าน) in Thailand.

This "thai villager research" cannot be reduced to participatory action research, like it was popular to do so in the 1980s and 1990s. Unlike this form of research, it is not initiated by Western researchers and development aid workers (e.g. western NGOs), but emerged from the need of local population groups themselves to improve their own living conditions and to exercise a knowledge-based critique of the activities of the central government in Bangkok. In this chapter, I will present both the emergence and the epistemic practice of "Thai Baan Research" and show to what extent its intersectional, intergenerational, transdisciplinary, and communal character might serve as a model for re-thinking how we produce scientific knowledge.

5.1   The Pak Mun Dam

From the mid-1980s to the early 2000s, Thailand experienced significant economic growth. A significant factor for this growth was the allocation and utilisation of the country's natural resources, especially its waterways. In the process, the interests of the central state were often placed above the needs of populations beyond the urbanised southern coast regions (Missingham 2003a, b). While the inequality between the rural and urban population of the country grew during the 1990s, the government started an initiative to gain energy independence from neighbouring countries. An essential building block for this project was to be the Pak Mun Dam (เขื่อนปากมูล) in the north-eastern Ubon Ratchathani province (อุบลราชธานี), which was built and inaugurated in the year 1994. The dam flooded immediately about 117 square kilometres of land and, contrary to original predictions, displaced 912 families, of which about 780 lost their agricultural livelihoods. Other social, economic and environmental consequences emerged in the years that followed its opening which, for many, far exceeded the dam's contribution to the country's energy supply. The affected families received rather insufficient reparations from the state (Kiguchi 2016). This concerned in particular those who were members of cultural and ethnic minority groups like the Sô or the Kui. These groups had been particularly "othered" by the mainstream society in Thailand and Laos both by antagonising and romanticising them (see Lamb 2018).

According to the political and environmental scientist Tun Myint, this governmental neglect lead to widespread protests among the rural population of Thailand (Myint 2016). The first step was to find ways for and by the rural communities to be heard in the capital. For this purpose, concerned individuals and groups across the country organised themselves in the so-called "Assembly of the Poor" (สมัชชาคนจน) a group that aimed to structure and unite the voices of the unheard populations and to demand a voice for them in policy decisions. These efforts included the occupation of the dam by 5000 villagers on 14 March 1999 to mark International Rivers Day, and a 99-day protest by 20,000 villagers in the capital (Missingham 2003a). The second step sought to generate media presence and to bring the concerns of the rural population into the public discourse in order to find supporters in the socially progressive circles of the urban groups and the international stage (Myint 2016). The third step, closely related to the previous two, was to link the villagers' own concern with a legitimising knowledge strategy. While the Thai government referred to expert opinions from universities and research institutions, emphasising in particular the global development benefits of the dam, the now organised villagers developed an alternative narrative that centred around their cultural perspectives and their experiential knowledge as a people who live with the rivers since countless generations. A central challenge to their endeavour, therefore, was a translational: "How can we, who are oftentimes pejoratively referred to as "uneducated water buffaloes" gain politically actionable epistemic authority?" (see Chainarong 2004). In other words, they aimed not only to voice their concerns but to become actionable against the backdrop of justified knowledge.

5.2   How to Do Science for the People by the People?

An opportunity for such villager research arose when Thaksin Shinawatra, the then popular political leader and prime minister, who particularly relied on the votes of rural regions, agreed to open the dam gates for four months in June 2001. Although this was only intended as an appeasing gesture of goodwill, the activists of the "Assembly of the Poor" seized their chance and began to outline a research plan for the social and ecological importance of the river.

The natural and cultural environment of the river, as well as its various forms of entanglement should be, according to the activists, explored from the perspective of local people's wisdom, their experiences, and their traditions. In order to achieve this goal, the village collectives started a collaboration with the Living River Siam project (โครงการแม่น้ำเพื่อชีวิต), founded at the peak of the protests in 1999. Given that the Thai government had commissioned classic research institutions to study the ecological impact of the dam, it became clear in the following months, that only the collaboration between the local population groups and the Living River Project was capable of meaningfully capturing the connection between the social reality and the ecological situation of life along the river (Ibid). Their Thai Baan approach connected narrative approaches towards local fishing traditions, gender roles, the use of plants and herbs, and the functional cycles of the various ecosystems along the river with both epidemiological and ecological data collection (Ibid). In this context, no form enquiry should be attributed with more importance over another from an epistemic perspective. Rather, the long-term self-directed observation led by the villagers themselves should generate a new, more localised but holistic form of valid knowledge (Lamb 2018).

To achieve this, the research was organised in a bottom-up manner. The sociologist Chainarong Sretthachau characterises the organisation, methodology and cooperation between villagers, the Living River Project and its partners in a short reflection from 2004 as follows:

> The methodology pays specific attention to including all villagers who are interested in engaging in the research- Villager researchers are selected by members of their own communities. Research teams are identified and involved in setting up their own terms of reference including collecting field data, taking samples and recording information based on their everyday local practices. With support from research assistants (…) the research findings are analysed (…). (Chainarong 2004)

A local villager and participant in Thai baan research additionally stated:

> We are the ones who suffer from all negative impacts (of the dam). We are the ones who are directly affected. Our lives have been destroyed by the dam, but when fish and nature are restored to the river, our lives are restored too. We are trying to make other people see and understand in the impacts of what has happened since the dam gates have been opened. And we thought of documenting the impacts of opening the dam gates by doing our own research. If outsiders conduct the research, we are afraid that they will not see the full picture, and will not consider all issues of the impacts from the dam because they are outsiders who live in cities and do not understand our lives. They do not know about fish, the ecosystem, and the Mun River like we do. Therefore, we decided to do our own research. (cited after: Myint 2016)

Control over the research is, in such a setting, designed to remain in the hands of the villagers. Their perspectival knowledge, or as feminist scholars might say "situated knowledge", must not be suppressed or silenced but rather brought into conversation with other forms of knowledge production (Pomun 2010). This finds a practical expression, for example, in the role that the creation and dissemination of topographical representations gained in Thai Baan research.

Spatial self-localisation is very important for many marginalised ethnic and cultural groups in Southeast Asia. The arbitrary borders that France drew in Southeast Asia during the colonial period which today separate todays nation states in no way represent the organically grown historical and spatial localisations of the people that lived and are still living in this region. Cultural belonging in Southeast Asia evolved alongside river systems such as the Chao Phraya (เจ้าพระยา), Mun (แม่น้ำมูล), Mekong (แม่น้ำโขง), or Salaween (แม่น้ำสาละวิน) and their respective environments. From a political perspective the opening of the Pak Mun Dam's sluice gates was connected to a symbolic re-examination of the connection between villager's livelihoods, industrial fisheries and the energy sector (Myint 2016) Yet, for the Thai baan researchers themselves, it opened the possibility to reconnect with their own collective identity. The river system environment that they might have taken for granted they now saw to be fragile due to the dam project. The fragility of the river system therefore became a reflection for the fragility of their social and cultural identity (Pomun 2010). To demonstrate the importance of the river, Thai Baan researchers began documenting both the return of human life and the restoration of different natural areas in the Mun River water system in August 2001. It was during the course of their enquiry, that they chose a geographical form to represent their findings and insights.

The maps that summarise their activities are highly inclusive with respect to different forms of knowledge. An epistemic hierarchisation between local knowledge, narrative accounts, quantified information, or other forms of enquiry is deliberately avoided. This applies both to the range of variation of the maps that emerged from the project and to the information that is summarised in the individual maps. The instrument of the map was chosen in a democratic voting process as an essential epistemic tool of the project because it can be used in an integrative way. As the project members explain, it is not difficult to draw a map. No special software, GPS or standard telemetry is needed, even though their use is not excluded. Basically, it would be enough to have a large sheet of paper that could be laid out on the village square or coloured chalk which allows every villager to draw and share her, his, or their knowledge and experiences (Watanaputi 2010) (see Figs. 5.1 and 5.2). The possibilities for participation in this way are extensive. What kind of water streams are there in the area? What trees grow here? Which animals live and lived in the observation area? Has their population suffered from the dam? What human settlements are nearby? What farming or fishing techniques are

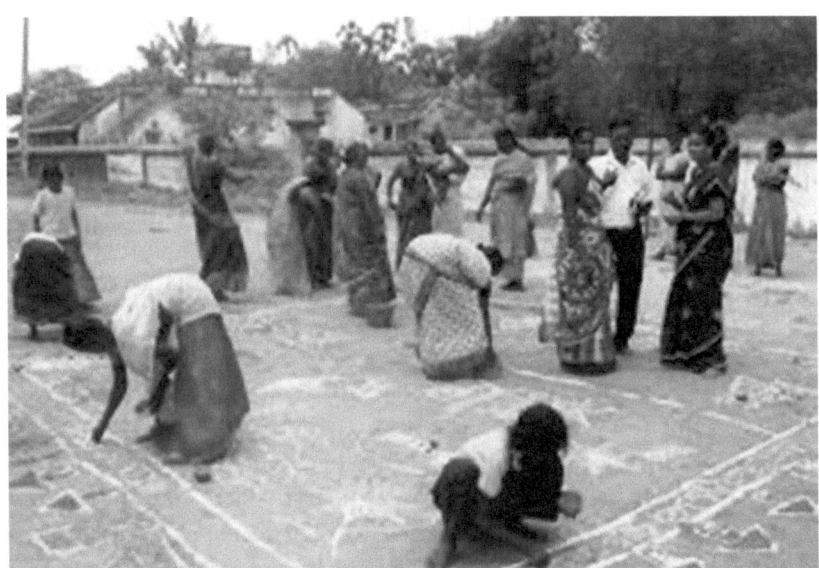

Fig. 5.1 Villagers in rural Thailand expressing their experiential knowledge about a local river system by drawing a map. (Source: http://developmentbloc. blogspot.com/2014/10/social-mapping.html?m=1)

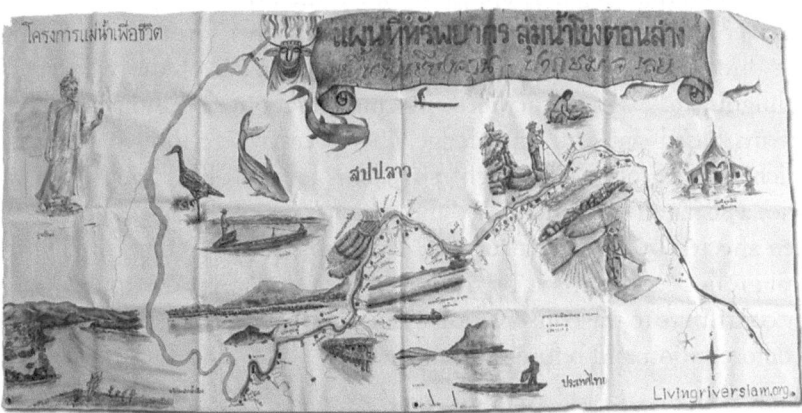

Fig. 5.2 Exemplary map of the Thai Baan research community. (Source: http:// developmentbloc.blogspot.com/2014/10/social-mapping.html?m=1)

used by yourself and other locals? What have you measured in the water, if you use such specialised methods, for example the concentration of microorganisms? Maps serve in this context as boundary objects, which are equally accessible for all involved actors. The sociological concept of boundary objects was introduced by Susan Leigh Star and James R. Griesemer (1989). It refers to objects that are used and interpreted in different ways by different people, that can acquire different meanings in different social worlds, but which are at the same time stable, accessible, and open enough for a wide variety of actors to participate in their production and use.

Even more elaborate maps were later used in negotiations with the Thai government and its appointed experts have an inclusive character. They do not hide the contribution of the village communities to the generation of knowledge about life in the Thai river systems, but rather integrate the knowledge expressed in their respective maps. An example of this is the ecosystem map of the Mekong basin area of Chaing Saen (เชียงแสน), Chiang Khong (เชียงของ) and Wiang Kaen (เวียงแก่น) districts of the Chiang Rai (เชียงราย) province presented in the final government audit of 2002 (Fig. 5.3).

Although this map may appear to be a standard GPS representation of the river basin, in reality it represents various other forms of knowledge that directly stem from the collaborative approach of the villagers. It highlights, for example, detailed information about 438 indigenous ecosystems based on local knowledge, the places where local people fish, which ethnic groups use which ecosystems for their livelihoods, the histories associated with the places and which parts of the river course have been affected by dam construction. The map also shows that some of the local groups characterised by the government as "forest destroyers" actually contribute to the conservation of local ecosystems in a specific rhythm of deforestation and reforestation.[1]

---

[1] However, as sociologist and geographer Vanessa Lamb points out in a gender-analytical contribution to lay river ecology research in Thailand and Myanmar, the distribution of tasks between the genders of the river dwellers is not sufficiently addressed in the Thai Baan representations. See: Lamb (2018).

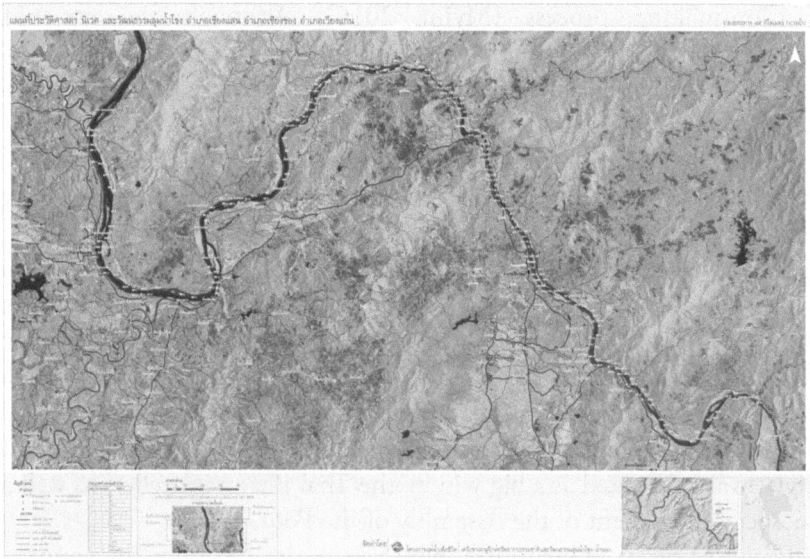

Fig. 5.3   Ecosystem map by the Thai Baan research community. (Source: http://www.livingriversiam.org/2work/tb/eco_map.html)

5.3   Alternative Knowledge and Political Empowerment

When the screening committee headed by the then Deputy Prime Minister Cavalit Yongchaiyudh met in January 2002 to review the results of the Pak Mun Dam research, Thai Baan research had become a media sensation in Thailand. Never before had Thai villagers conducted their own research to influence national policy decisions regarding the country's resources (Suwankhong and Liamputtong 2015). At the same time, some of the authors of one of the official research reports took an oppositional position towards the validity and reliability of the research conducted by the project (see: Kirchherr 2018). In the eyes of these experts, Thai Baan's integrative approach would not be very meaningful and would dilute scientific knowledge with individual opinions (see: Molle et al. 2009). Despite such criticisms, the screening committee decided to make the summary of the Thai Baan research one of four sources for its decision-making process (Myint 2016). Although the screening committee considered a study by Ubon Ratchathani University (มหาวิทยาลัย อุบลราชธานี) to be the most meaningful, the knowledge of the Thai Baan Report, co-produced by local communities, was also taken seriously by the assembled decision-makers because the studies of the lay researchers and their specific experiential expertise were shown to complement the university report in many ways. Together, they painted a cohesive picture of the convergence of indigenous lifestyles and agricultural practices, as well as the ecological richness of the countries riverine regions. On this basis, the audit panel decided to advise the Prime Minister of the country that the dam gates should remain open for most of the year. This should allow local communities to maintain their culture while preserving the identity and ecological richness of Thailand's river basins. The audits advise was celebrated as a big win by the Thai Baan researchers as well as the social movement of the Assembly of the Poor.

Prime Minister Shinawantra, who was under fire from the country's economic and royal elites at the time, found himself in a dilemma over this advice. In order to maintain his political influence, he had to reach a compromise, even though he had originally supported the villagers' concerns through the media. According to Tun Myint, the prime minister met on December 20, 2002 with 30 representatives of villagers and the University's research team. This encounter was even broadcasted live on major television channels and accompanied by documentaries about Thai Baan activities and the lives of the population groups living in the region of the Mun river. Shinawantra even agreed to visit some of the villages personally and then to make an appropriate decision (Ibid). In the coming weeks, nonetheless, the Prime Minister commissioned (in an ad hoc manner) further studies on the situation. This time, however, no research institutions or local stakeholders were involved, but the Second Army, the Border Police and the National Bureau of Statistics. Based on their reports as well as a consensus of the university and Thai Baan reports, it was finally decided on 14 January to keep the gates of the dam open for four months each year.

5.4   Conclusion

Although the final decision by the Thai government was ultimately rather disappointing for the indigenous peoples of the river basin, from a meta-perspective, it can also be seen as a success. Never before had the knowledge of the rural poor been taken so seriously as a decision-making factor in Thai society. The example of activism against the Mun River Dam has changed this (Ibid). Implicit, local and experiential knowledge was valorised nationwide, and the spatial methods of lay cartographic research even became an intellectual import in the years to come, used in Vietnam and China, among other places (LRA 2020).

Such epistemic strategies give underrepresented groups the opportunity to draw attention to their own concerns in a "language" that can be easily translated into scientific and political discourse. This creates a form of empowerment of marginalised populations based on a certain epistemic authority. At the same time, the Thai Baan research also shows that a problem-centred collection and dissemination of local knowledge can have an identity-creating or identity-affirming function. The bottom-up organised villager research ultimately transformed marginalised groups into actors with a certain socio-political influence. At the same time, it reinforced a sense of belonging, in this case less oriented towards the Thai nation-state but rather as members of cultural groups who see the country's river systems as their habitat and want to preserve their ecology. For them, it is not state borders that create identity, but the branched, complex and variable structure of the waterways. This, I believe, is the unique power of collectively generated knowledge that is based on experiences: it focuses on the needs of real people and is oriented towards finding solutions for their problems. Epistemic ingenuity, and the use of the knowledge it produces may be understood from this perspective as something of an anthropological constant. Herein, the Thai Baan approach resembles social health movements of the 1970s. The forms of engagement, knowledge production, and the villager's protest are very similar to the way in which poor Americans exercised their agency in the case of toxic waste dumps in Woburn, Massachusetts.

In 1972, a resident of Woburn whose son was just diagnosed with acute leukaemia suspected that the cause lay in the water contamination by nearby factories. She began collecting evidence from other residents, often women, and, with the help of a pastor, helped organise the community. Although the state department in charge of water quality was well aware of toxic levels in the river since at least 1972, the information did not reach the public. In 1979, a chance discovery of almost 200 chemical barrels containing an unknown substance along the river, and close to two wells where drinking water was pumped, confirmed the public's suspicion about the water quality, which tasted and smelled bad. In the following years, residents engaged in what the historian Phil Brown calls "popular epidemiology" (Brown 1997), collecting and analysing experiential data about resident health and its possible connection to water contamination. Popular epidemiology is not just classical epidemiology performed with the help of lay people. It broadens the spectra of causative agents, including social factors, and challenges traditional assumptions about risk analysis, such as dose-response relationships. Yet, in the cases studied by Brown, lay people worked together with professional epidemiologists, uniting "lay and professional perspectives in an effort to link science and politics" (Ibid). Together, they identified a cluster of leukaemia that could be linked to the contaminated water, by conducting interviews of residents about pregnancies and child disorders for example. The residents' study, eventually supported by Harvard public health and epidemiology experts, formed the evidential basis for the litigation against the two companies that had leaked toxic waste in the water.

But the residents' opposition was also directed towards state scientists who ignored, minimised, or omitted evidence of contamination. Physicians also offered limited support to residents, at least in the early history of toxic waste mobilisation, because they tended to explain away the occurrence of diseases through biological, and not environmental, causes This only reinforced the community's attempts to rely on their own experiential knowledge rather than on state experts. As Brown notes, "residents begin to distrust traditional scientific authorities when those authorities contradict the experiential knowledge the community has gathered and developed" (Ibid). Although the outcome of the trial was only a modest victory for the plaintiffs, it helped establish a model, discussed in the media nationwide, of how residents could produce scientific knowledge about their health and environment. As Brown put it, "the popular epidemiological approach to toxic waste contamination in Woburn and other toxic waste sites gives much more credibility and power to the lay public than does the governmental version of public participation" (Ibid). Both, the example of the resistance towards the Pan Mun Dam and popular epidemiology in Woburn emphasise the timeless character of local experiential knowledge as a form of epistemic counter expertise.

References

Brown, Phil. 1997. "Popular Epidemiology" Revisited. *Current Sociology* 45 (3): 137–156.

Chainarong, Sretthachau. 2004. *Case Study for Empowerment and Democratisation High Level Panel.* http://www.livingriversiam.org/2work/tb/tb_a7.html. Accessed 9 Dec 2020.

Kiguchi, Yuk. 2016. Pak Moon Dam Still a Dilemma 25 Years On. *Bangkok Post* (online). https://www.bangkokpost.com/opinion/opinion/872044/pak-moon-dam-still-a-dilemma-25-years-on. Accessed 18 Dec 2020.

Kirchherr, Julian. 2018. Strategies of Successful Anti-Dam Movements: Evidence from Myanmar and Thailand. *Society & Natural Resources* 31 (2): 166–182.

Lamb, Vanessa. 2018. Who Knows the River? Gender, Expertise, and the Politics of Local Ecological Knowledge Production of the Salween River, Thai-Myanmar Border. *Gender, Place & Culture* 25 (12): 1703–1718.

LRA. Living River Association. 2020. *Training and Enhancing the Thai Baan Research Network. Both Domestic and International.* http://www.livingriversiam.org/our-work?view=article&id=32:tbr-training&catid=32:taibaan. Accessed 18 Dec 2020.

Missingham, Bruce D. 2003a. *The Environmental Evaluation on Social and Economic Conditions of the Population Receiving Impact on Housing: Pak Man Hydropower Project.* Final Report. http://mrcmekong.org/assets/Consultations/LuangPrabang-Hydropower-Project/LPHPP_PNPCA-Report_Vol-4-Part-1-of-3Marked.pdf. Accessed 18 Dec 2020.

————. 2003b. Forging Solidarity and Identity in the Assembly of the Poor. From Local Struggle to National Social Movement in Thailand. *Asian Studies Review* 27 (3): 317–340.

Molle, Francois, Tira Foran, and Mira Käkönen, eds. 2009. *Contested Waterscapes in the Mekong Region. Hydropower, Livelihoods and Governance.* London: Earthscan.

Myint, Tun. 2016. *Citizen Science in a Democracy: The Case of Thai Baan Research.* Tocquevill Lecture. https://ostromworkshop.indiana.edu/pdf/seriespapers/2016F_Tocq/Myint%20paper.pdf. Accessed 25 July 2021.

Pomun, Teerapong. 2010. *Local Knowledge and Food Security in the Mekong River Basin.* http://www.livingriversiam.org/2work/tb/tb_a8.pdf. Accessed 18 Dec 2020.

Star, Susan Leigh, and R. James. 1989. Institutional Ecology, "Translations" and Boundary Objects: Amateurs and Professionals in Berkeley's Museum of Vertebrate Zoology, 1907–39. *Social Studies of Science* 19 (3): 387–420.

Stollberg, Gunnar. 2001. *Medizinsoziologie. Einsichten,* Themen der Soziologie. Bielefeld: Transcript.

Suwankhong, Dusanee, and Pranee Liamputtong. 2015. Cultural Insiders and Research Fieldwork: Case Examples from Cross-Cultural Research with Thai People. *International Journal of Qualitative Methods* 14 (5). https://doi.org/10.1177/2F1609406915621404. Accessed 18 Dec 2020.

Watanaputi, Chayan. 2010. *Thai Baan Research Community Research for Community.* http://www.livingriversiam.org/2work/tb/tb_a2.html. Accessed 18 Dec 2020.

6

Summary

Abstract How can we shape science differently in the twenty-first century? Against the backdrop of the three case studies (Chaps. 3, 4 and 5) this final chapter revisits current forms of science education and participatory knowledge production (e.g. citizen science and open science) and develops a roadmap towards a more inclusive, diverse, and human science beyond mere social representation and tokenism.

Keywords Open science • Citizen science • Participatory knowledge production • Diversity in science

"Follow the Science, listen to the experts, do what they tell you", this appeal to the public by then presidential candidate Joe Biden during an interview with the ABC news-anchor George Stephanopoulos in April 2020 testifies that he is both scientifically informed and able to take responsibility (ABC News 2020). In an ideal world where epistemic knowledge might be free of values and is accepted by every individual, Biden's words would probably have led to a quick end of the Covid19 pandemic. In the reality of the year 2020 (and most likely far 2021) the end of the pandemic will be different and more complicated. Everyone would wear face masks, observe the rules of social distancing and within a month the nightmare would probably be over. The knowledge and expertise of scientists and responsible decision-makers would be heard because they would largely speak only with one voice.

Science as a practice is not to be equated with such an idealistic idea of science. In this book, I have shown how the production of scientific knowledge is human and arbitrary: it is historically, socially, and culturally situated. I have also shown how this human side of science has contributed to a loss of trust in various knowledge-based institutions and which institutional strategies are being used to counter this loss of trust. Programmes such as citizen science or open science represent an attempt to reconnect the sciences with the general public, communicating participation in the production of knowledge as a panacea. In this way, however, science reaches only a fraction of society and reproduces traditional power structures on a social and epistemic level. Most digital citizen science projects make use of a top-down organisation and clearly distributed roles. The scientists at the top of the project specify what will be researched, what methods will be used, and make their judgement on what contribution is relevant. The participating volunteers, on the other hand, are given limited, predefined tasks and are turned into (unpaid) helpers. To what extent this can contribute to a better understanding of science or to political empowerment of the participants in such projects is still an open question (Mahr et al. 2018). It is therefore not surprising that alternative epistemic movements are emerging beyond this instrumental form of "democratisation of knowledge".

These social movements and the knowledge they produce pose a great challenge to institutional science. The instinctive reaction of many proponents of scientific knowledge, such as Richard Dawkins, is to be sceptical and combative towards alternative forms of knowledge. The fear of so-called pseudosciences is so deeply rooted that the institution of science often even deprives itself of the possibility of receiving new stimuli from outsiders. It therefore seems more important too many popularisers of science to assert and defend the vision of a unity of science than to embrace the reality of epistemic plurality. Almost all alternative epistemological strategies are equated with anti-vaccinationists, flat-earthers, or neo-creationists and dismissed as either a danger or ridiculous behaviour by a few deluded individuals. But like other alternative epistemic movements, these extreme groups are not so much proponents of a danger as they are an expression of the aforementioned loss of trust. Of course, restoring confidence in the sciences is one response to this loss. But the important question is: how?

One way of restoring trust has a didactic character. Science in the twenty-first century should understand its own heterogeneity as a strength and communicate it to the public. A plural world needs a plural science and not the caricature of an epistemic unity. This is a challenge for the education system, for the training of young scientists as well as for science communication. The second way, both systemic and complementary, is to take seriously the concerns of alternative epistemic movements. Can their methods and views perhaps even broaden the perspective on what "good science" can be? The three case studies I have presented in this book give an indication for the possibility to renew the institution of science from the societal margins. Trust does not arise from delegating partial aspects of scientific activity to the public, but from giving the public the opportunity to generate knowledge on their own responsibility, which reflects their life situation. Science can thus become more multifaceted and better reflect reality, for example in the field of medicine, and perhaps even rediscover itself epistemically.

Although they emerged from entirely different context, the "alternative epistemic communities" presented in the three case studies of this book have much in common. The online support groups of people with inflammatory bowel diseases, the new radical women's health movements with their DIY practices, as well as the Thai Baan research emerged from a need to challenge concrete social inequalities. These inequalities are directly experienced by them, be it in terms of insecurities about the use of health information through commercial health platforms, the prevailing marginalisation of some women in medicine, or the threat to one's own cultural and natural environment in north-west Thailand. Unlike flat-earthers or anti-vaccinationists, they also address with their activities concrete adversaries: commercial providers of online self-help structures, non-inclusive health care systems, and the environmental policies of the Thai government. In the debate with these actors, they claim a knowledge advantage. Unlike the institutional experts many decision-makers rely on, they operationalise their own experience as an epistemic resource. What does it mean to live with a chronic illness, to be perceived as a second-class citizen in the health system, or to lose one's livelihood? Only personally affected individuals and social groups can find a valid and good answer to such questions and share them with others. It is also important to communicate this knowledge strategically and coherently, both internally and to potential allies or opponents. The success of the social epistemic movements I studied was therefore based on the establishment of epistemic objects and strategies that are internally inclusive and externally coherent. The best example of this is the topographical, geographical approach of the researching villagers of the Thai Baan movement. They collectively translate their experiences of the river flows of Thailand and the cultural traditions based on them into a medium that can also be understood in the social systems of science or politics. The same applies to the meticulously conducted statistical studies of the menstrual cycle by members of the women's health movement and the peer-controlled DIY faecal transplants by patients with Crohn's disease and ulcerative colitis. The aim is not so much to pursue a "counter-science", but to generate complementary knowledge, which on the one hand underlines one's own concerns and experiences, but on the other hand should also add a new facet to the knowledge of science. In other words, they invite institutional science to expand its epistemic toolbox to include experiential knowledge by the people and for the people.

The task of a self-aware and open science will therefore be to integrate such knowledge in a non-hegemonic or reductionist form. Perhaps in this way some of those who feel alienated from science may even be won back. Trust arises neither via tokenism nor by being involved in the solution of prefabricated tasks, but by meeting other people where they stand.

References

ABC News. 2020. Joe Biden Answers How he Would Have Handled the Pandemic. https://abcnews.go.com/Politics/video/joe-biden-answers-handled-pandemic-73643459. Accessed 25 July 2021.

Mahr, Dana, Claudia Göbel, Alan Irwin, and Katrin Vohland. 2018. Watching or Being Watched – Enhancing Productive Discussion Between the Citizen Sciences, the Social Sciences and the Humanities. In *Citizen Science: Innovation in Open Science, Society and Policy*, ed. Susanne Hecker, Muki Haklay, Anne Bowser, Zen Makuch, and Johannes Vogel. London: UCL Press. https://doi.org/10.14324.

References

ABC News. 2020. *Joe Biden Answers How he Would Have Handled the Pandemic.* https://abcnews.go.com/Politics/video/joe-biden-answers-handled-pandemic-73643459. Accessed 25 July 2021.

Adams, Patrick. 2020. Amid Covid-19, a Call for M.D.s or Mail the Abortion Pill. *The New York Times* (online). https://www.nytimes.com/2020/05/12/opinion/covid-abortion-pill.html. Visited 25 May 2020. https://doi.org/10.1098/rstb.2013.0152

Alvarez-Salvado, Efren, Vincente Pallares, Andrea Moreno, and Santiago Canals. 2014. Functional MRI of Long-Term Potentiation: Imaging Network Plasticity. *Philosophical Transactions of the Royal Society B* 369 (1633). https://doi.org/10.1098/rstb.2013.0152.

Atarashi, Koji, Takeshi Tanoue, Tatsuichiro Shima, Akemi Imaoka, Tomomi Kuwahara, Yoshika Momose, Genhong Cheng, Sho Yamasaki, Takashi Saito, Yusuke Ohba, Tadatsugu Taniguchi, Kiyoshi Takeda, Shohei Hori, Ivaylo I. Ivanov, Yoshinori Umesaki, Kikuji Ithoh, and Keny Honda. 2011. Induction of Colonic Regulatory T Cells by Indigenous Clostridium Species. *Science* 331 (6015): 337–341. https://doi.org/10.1126/science.1198469. Accessed 6 Apr 2020.

Atienza, Milagros F., Ronald T. Burkman, Theodore M. King, Lonnie S. Burnett, H. Lorrin Lau, Tim H. Parmley, and J. Donald Woodruff. 1975. Menstrual Extraction. *American Journal of Obstetrics and Gynecology* 121 (4): 490–495. https://doi.org/10.1016/0002-9378(75)90080-0. Accessed 6 Apr 2020.

Banner, Olivia. 2017. *Communicative Biocapitalism*. Arbor: Michigan Publishing.

Bass, Emily, Burns Julien, and Deidre Grant. 2013. Citizen Scientists and Activist Researchers: Building and Sustaining HIV Prevention Research Advocacy in the Era of Evidence. In *Global HIV/AIDS Politics, Policy, and Activism, 3: Activism and Community Mobilization*, ed. A. Raymond, 135–156. Santa Barbara: Praeger.

Bauer, Jared (Wisecrack). 2019. *Flat Earth: What Makes REAL Science - Wiserack Edition. Youtube Video Essay*. https://www.youtube.com/watch?v=umo6pMCkcXs. Accessed 25 July 2021.

Baxandall, Rosalyn, and Linda Gordon. 2020. *Dear Sisters. Dispatches form the Women's Liberation Movement*. New York: Basic Books.

Beck, Ulrich. 2003 (=1986). *Risikogesellschaft*. Frankfurt a. M.: Suhrkamp.

Belluck, Pam. 2020. Abortion by Telemedicine: A Growing Option as Access to Clinics Wanes. *The Guardian* (online). https://www.nytimes.com/2020/04/28/health/telabortion-abortion-telemedicine.html?referringSource=articleShare. Accessed 26 May 2020.

Benkler, Yochai. 2006. *The Wealth of Networks: How Social Production Transforms Markets and Freedom*. New Haven: Yale University Press.

Bierend, Dough. 2015. Meet the GynePunks Pushing the Boundaries of DIY Gynecology. *Motherboard* (online). http://motherboard.vice.com/read/meet-the-gynepunks-pushing-the-boundaries-of-diy-gynecology. Accessed 18 Dec 2020.

Bleker, Johanna. 1998. *Der Eintritt der Frauen in die Gelehrtenrepublik. Zur Geschlechterfrage im akademischen Selbstverständnis und in der wissenschaftlichen Praxis am Anfang des 20. Jahrhunderts*. Abhandlungen zur Geschichte der Medizin und der Naturwissenschaften 84. Husum: Matthiesen.

Boston Women's Health Collective. 1970. *Women and Their Bodies: A Course*. Boston: BWHC.

Boyle, Peter, Nigel Gray, Jack Henningfield, John Seffrin, and Witold A. Zatonski, eds. 2010. *Tobacco. Science, Policy, and Public Health*. 2nd ed. Oxford: Oxford University Press.

Bracher, Karl-Dietrich. 1969. *Die deutsche Diktatur: Entstehung, Struktur, Folgen des Nationalsozialismus*. Köln: Kieenheuer & Witsch.

Bradbury-Jones, Caroline, and Louise Isham. 2020. The Pandemic Paradox: The Consequences of COVID-19 on Domestic Violence. *Journal of Clinical Nursing. Early View.* https://doi.org/10.1111/jocn.15296.

Braveman, Paula. 2010. Social Conditions, Health Equity, and Human Rights. *Health Human Rights* 12 (2): 31–48. PMID: 21178188.

Brewis, Harry (@hbomberguy). 2019. Flat Earth: A Measured Response. *YouTube.* www.youtube.com/watch?v=2gFsOoKAHZg. Accessed 9 Dec 2020.

Brown, Phil. 1997. "Popular Epidemiology" Revisited. *Current Sociology* 45 (3): 137–156.

Brubaker, Jed, Caitlin Lustig, and Gillian R. Hayes. 2020. *PatientsLikeMe: Empowerment and Representation in a Patient-Centered Social Network.* https://www.semanticscholar.org/paper/PatientsLikeMe-%3A-Empowerment-and-Representation-in-Brubaker-Lustig/1917dcade334dba9 1f15f9fdb259e7c128374151. Accessed 30 Dec 2020.

Bynum, William F. 1994. *Science and the Practice of Medicine in the Nineteenth Century.* Cambridge: Cambridge University Press.

Bynum, William F., Anne Hardy, Stephen Jacyna, Christopher Lawrence, and E.M. Tilli. 2006. *The Western Medical Tradition. 1800 to 2000.* Cambridge: Cambridge University Press.

Callon, Michel, and Rabeharisoa Vololona. 2007. The Growing Engagement of Emergent Concerned Groups in Political and Economic Life: Lessons from the French Association of Neuromuscular Disease Patients. *Science, Technology, & Human Values* 33 (2): 230–261.

Carpenter, Morgan. 2018. Intersex Variations, Human Rights, and the International Classification of Diseases. *Health and Human Rights* 20 (2): 205–214.

Casilli, Antonio A., and Julian Posada Gutierrez. 2019. The Platformization of Labor and Society. In *Society and the Internet*, ed. M. Graham and W.H. Dutton, 2nd ed., 293–306. Oxford University Press.

Casola, Valentina, Aniello Castiglione, Raymond Choo Kim-Kwang, and Christian Esposito. 2016. *Healthcare-Related Data in the Cloud: Challenges and Opportunities.* https://doi.org/10.1109/MCC.2016.139. Accessed 9 Dec 2020.

Chainarong, Sretthachau. 2004. *Case Study for Empowerment and Democratisation High Level Panel.* http://www.livingriversiam.org/2work/tb/tb_a7.html. Accessed 9 Dec 2020.

Chalker, Rebecca. 1993. The Whats, Hows, and Whys of Menstrual Extraction. *On the Issues* 26: 42–55.

Chardronnet, Ewen. 2015. GynePunk, the Cyborg Witches of DIY Gynecology. *Makery* (online). http://www.makery.info/en/2015/06/30/gynepunk-les-sorcieres-cyborg-de-la-gynecologie-diy/. Accessed 9 Dec 2020.

Chateuvert, Melinda. 2013. *Sex Workers Unite. A History of the Movement from Stonewall to Slut Walk*. Boston: Beacon Press.

ChoGlueck, Christopher. 2017. *What Are Scientific Facts? ScIU Conversations in Science at Indiana University*. https://blogs.iu.edu/sciu/2017/10/31/what-are-scientific-facts/. Accessed 9 Dec 2020.

Cole, Jennifer, Jason Nolan, Yukari Seko, Katherine Mancuso, and Alejandra Ospina. 2011. GimpGirl Grows Up: Women with Disabilities Rethinking, Redefining, and Reclaiming Community. *New Media & Society* 13 (7): 1161–1179.

Collins, Harry. 2015. *Are We All Scientific Experts Now?* Boston: Polity Press.

Colonia ecoindustrial postcapitalista. 2014. *A TransHackFeminist (THF!) Convergence Report from Calafou*. https://calafou.org/en/content/transhackfeminist-thf-convergence-report. Accessed 9 Dec 2020.

Conrad, Peter, and Cheryl Stults. 2010. The Internet and the Experience of Illness. In *Handbook of Medical Sociology*, 179–191. Nashville: Vanderbilt University Press.

Crohn's and Colitis UK. 2015. *Crohn's and Colitis Awareness*. https://www.facebook.com/CrohnsColitisAwareness/posts/890843521000986. Accessed 9 Dec 2020.

Crohnology. 2020. https://crohnology.com/. Accessed 9 Dec 2020.

Daston, Lorraine. 2001. Objektivität und die Flucht aus der Perspektive. In *Wunder, Beweise und Tatsachen. Zur Geschichte der Rationalität*, ed. Lorraine Daston, 127–156. Frankfurt a. M.: Fischer.

Daston, Lorraine, and Peter Galison. 2010. *Objectivity*. Cambridge: Zone Books.

Dawkins, Richard. 2015. Is It a Theory? *Is It a Law? No, It's A Fact*. https://www.richarddawkins.net/2015/11/is-it-a-theory-is-it-a-law-no-its-a-fact/. Accessed 9 Dec 2020.

DCCV e.V. 2020. *Wir Über Uns*. https://www.dccv.de/die-dccv/wir-ueber-uns/. Accessed 9 Dec 2020.

DCCV-Forum. 2014. *Thema Genetik*. https://forum.dccv.de/viewtopic.php?f=3&t=1806. Accessed 9 Dec 2020.

De Lauretis, Teresa. 1990. Upping the Anti in Feminist Theory. In *Conflicts in Feminism*, ed. Marianne Hirsch and Evelyn Fox Keller, 255–270. London: Routledge.

Delfanti, Alessandro. 2013. *Biohackers. The Politics of Open Science*. London: Pluto Press.

Dubriwny, Tasha N. 2013. *The Vulnerable Empowered Woman: Feminism, Postfeminism, and Women's Health*, Critical Issues in Health and Medicine. New Brunswick: Rutgers University Press.

Dupuy, Beatrice, and Jude Joffe-Block. 2020. Video Contains a Litany of False Claims About COVID-19 and Vaccines. *AP News*, December 10. https://apnews.com/article/fact-checking-afs:Content:9837440018. Accessed 9 Dec 2020.

Ehrenreich, Barbara. 1984. Body Politic: The Growth of the Women's Health Movement. *Ms. Magazine*. http://www.msmagazine.com/spring2002/ehrenreichandfuntes.asp. Accessed 9 Dec 2020.

Ehrlich, Paul, and Rudolph Gonder. 1914. *Experimentelle Chemotherapie*. https://www.pei.de/SharedDocs/Downloads/DE/institut/veroeffentlichungen-von-paul-ehrlich/1906-1914/1914-experimentelle-chemotherapie.pdf?__blob=publicationFile&v=2. Accessed 9 Dec 2020.

Elkeles, Barbara. 1996. *Der moralische Diskurs über das medizinische Menschenexperiment im 19. Jahrhundert*. Stuttgart: Fischer.

Epstein, Steven. 1995. The Construction of Lay Expertise: AIDS Activism and the Forging of Credibility in the Reform of Clinical Trials. *Science, Technology, & Human Values* 20 (4): 408–437.

European Parliament. P8_TA(2019)0111. 2019. *Experiencing Backlash in Women's Rights and Gender Equality in the EU*. http://www.europarl.europa.eu/doceo/document/TA-8-2019-0111_EN.html. Accessed 9 Dec 2020.

Fausto-Sterling, Anne. 1993. The Five Sexes: Why Male and Female Are Not Enough. *The Sciences* 33 (2).: 20p.

———. 2012. *Sex/Gender. Biology in a Social World*. New York: Routledge.

Fausto-Sterling, Anne, and Edward Stein. 2004 (=2000). *Sexing the Body: Gender Politics and the Construction of Sexuality*. New York: Basic Books.

FFWHC – Federation of Feminist Women's Health Centers. 1991. *A New View of a Woman's Body. A Fully Illustrated Guide*. 10th anniversary ed. West Hollywood: Feminist Health Press.

Fiske, Amelia, Lorenzo del Savio, Barbara Prainsack, and Alena Buyx. 2018. Conceptual and Ethical Considerations for Citizen Science in Biomedicine. In *Personal Health Science*, ed. Nils Heyen, Sascha Dickel, and Anne Brüninghaus, 195–217. München: Springer.

Fleck, Ludwik. 2017 (=1935). *Entstehung und Entwicklung einer wissenschaftlichen Tatsache*, Frankfurt a. M.: Suhrkamp.

Fornai, Francesco, Patrizia Longone, Luisa Camaro, Olga Kastsichuenka, Michaela Ferrucci, Michaela Laura Manca, Gloria Lazzeri, Alida Spalloni, Nastacia Bellio, Paola Lenzu, Gabriele Modugno, Isodoro Siciliano, Murri

Ciro, Stefano Ruggieri, and Antonio Paparelli. 2008. Lithium Delays Progression of Amyotrophic Lateral Sclerosis. *Oric National Academy of Sciences USA* 105 (6): 16404–16407.

Foucault, Michel, and Colin Gordon. 1980. *Power/Knowledge: Selected Interviews and Other Writings 1972–1977*. New York: Vintage Books.

Frankfort, Ellen. 1972. *Vaginal Politics. Who Controls a Woman's Body: Doctors? Lovers? Drugs? Women?* New York: Bantam Books.

———. 1973. Medicine, the Feminist Frontier. *The New York Times*, March 3.

Garcia-Sanjuan, Sofia, Manuel Lillo-Crespo, Angela Sanjuan-Quiles, Diana Gil-Gonzales, and Miguel Richart-Martinez. 2016. Life Experiences of People Affected by Crohn's Disease and Their Support Networks: Scoping Review. *Clinical Nursing Research* 25 (1): 79–99.

Gender and Covid-19. 2020. *Open Mendely Group Initiated by Rosemary Morgan.* https://www.mendeley.com/community/gender-and-covid-19/. Accessed 9 Dec 2020.

Green, Eli R. 2006. Debating Transw Inclusion in the Feminist Movement. A Trans-Positive Analysis. *Journal of Lesbian Studies* 10 (1–2): 231–248.

Greshake Tzovaras, Bastian. 2020. *E-Mail – Bastian Greshake Tzovaras and Dana Mahr*, January 7. https://outlook.unige.ch/owa/#path=/mail. Accessed 9 Dec 2020.

Grosberg, Dafna, Haya Grinvald, Haim Reuveni, and Racheli Magnezi. 2016. Frequent Surfing on Social Health Networks is Associated with Increased Knowledge and Patient Health Activation. *Journal of Medical Internet Research* 18 (8). https://doi.org/10.2196/jmir.5832. Accessed 9 Dec 2020.

harpgirl. 2012. Menstrual Extractions: Controversy and Safety. *Social Health Network. Political Mingling (PLM Forum)*, August 24. https://www.patientslikeme.com/forum/ms/topics/102276?post_id=1759024#post-1759024. Accessed 9 Dec 2020.

Hecker, Susanne, Rick Bonney, Muki Haklay, and Franz Hölker, eds. 2018. Innovation in Citizen Science – Perspectives on Science-Policy Advances. *Citizen Science: Theory and Practice* 3 (1). https://doi.org/10.5334/cstp.114. Accessed 9 Dec 2020.

Heffernan, Virginia. 2011. Online Medical Advice Can Be a Prescription for Fear. *The New York Times*, February 4, sec. Magazine. https://www.nytimes.com/2011/02/06/magazine/06FOB-Medium-t.html. Accessed 9 Dec 2020.

Hekman, Susan. 1997. Truth and Method: Feminist Standpoint Theory Revisited. *Signs* 22 (2): 341–365.

Herrn, Rainer. 2005. *Schnittmuster des Geschlechts. Transvestitismus und Transsexualität in der frühen Sexualwissenschaft*. Gießen: Psychosozial-Verlag.

Hodgson, Jane E. 1974. Menstrual Extraction: Putting It and All It's Synonyms into Proper Perspective as Pseudonyms. *JAMA* 228 (7): 849. https://doi.org/10.1001/jama.1974.03230320019018. Accessed 9 Dec 2020.

Hoesch, Kristin. 1995. *Ärztinnen für Frauen. Kliniken in Berlin 1877–1914.* Stuttgart/Weimar: Metzler.

Hoffman, Lily M. 1982. *The Politics of Knowledge. Activist Movements in Medicine and Planning.* New York: State University of New York Press.

Høivik, Marte Lee, Tomm Bernklev, Inger Camilla Solberg, Milada Cvancarova, Ida Lygren, Jørgen Jahnsen, and Bjørn Moum. 2012. The IBSEN Study Group, Patients with Crohn's Disease Experience Reduced General Health and Vitality in the Chronic Stage: Ten-Year Results from the IBSEN Study. *Journal of Crohn's and Colitis* 6 (4): 441–453. https://doi.org/10.1016/j.crohns.2011.10.001. Accessed 18 Dec 2020.

Hollander, Judd E., and Brendan G. Carr. 2020. Virtually Perfect? Telemedicine for Covid-19. *The New England Journal of Medicine* 382: 1679–1681. https://doi.org/10.1056/NEJMp2003539.

Huh, Jina, Rebecca Marmor, and Xiaoqian Jiang. 2016. Lessons Learned for Online Health Community Moderator Roles: A Mixed-Methods Study of Moderators Resigning from WebMD Communities. *Journal of Medical Internet Research* 18 (9): e247. https://doi.org/10.2196/jmir.6331. Accessed 18 Dec 2020.

IPCC. 2014. *AR5 Climate Change 2014: Impacts, Adaption, and Vulnerability.* https://www.ipcc.ch/report/ar5/wg2/. Accessed 18 Dec 2020.

Irigaray, Luce. 1985. *Speculum of the Other Woman.* Ithaca: Cornell University Press.

Janssens, A., J.W. Cecile, and Peter Kraft. 2012. Research Conducted Using Data Obtained Through Online Communities: Ethical Implications of Methodological Limitations. *PloS Med* 9 (10): e1001328.

Jen, Clare. 2015. Do-It-Yourself Biology, Garage Biology, and Kitchen Science – A Feminist Analysis of Bio-Making Narratives. In *Knowing New Biotechnologies: Social Aspects of Technological Convergence, Genetics and Society*, ed. Matthias Wienroth and Eugenia Rorigues, 125–141. London/New York: Routledge/Taylor & Francis Group.

Jordanova, Ludmilla. 1989. *Sexual Visions. Images of Gender in Science and Medicine Between the Eighteenth and Twentieth Centuries.* Madison: University of Wisconsin Press.

Kalafateli, Maria, Christos Triantos, Georgios Theocharis, Dimitra Giannakopoulou, Efstratios Koutroumpakis, Chronis Aristidis, Apostolos Sapountzis Vasileios Margaritis, Konstantinos Thomopoulos, and Vasiliki

Nikolopoulou. 2013. Health-Related Quality of Life in Patients with Inflammatory Bowel Disease: A Single-Center Experience. *Annals of Gastroenterology* 26 (3): 243–248.

Katrini, Eleni. 2018. Sharing Culture: On Definitions, Values, and Emergence. *The Sociological Review* 66 (2): 425–446. https://doi. org/10.1177/0038026118758550. Accessed 18 Dec 2020.

Kiguchi, Yuk. 2016. Pak Moon Dam Still a Dilemma 25 Years On. *Bangkok Post* (online). https://www.bangkokpost.com/opinion/opinion/872044/pak-moon-dam-still-a-dilemma-25-years-on. Accessed 18 Dec 2020.

Kirchherr, Julian. 2018. Strategies of Successful Anti-Dam Movements: Evidence from Myanmar and Thailand. *Society & Natural Resources* 31 (2): 166–182.

Kullenberg, Christopher, and Dick Kasperowski. 2016. What Is Citizen Science? – A Scientometric Meta-Analysis. *PLoS One* 11 (1): e0147152. https://doi.org/10.1371/journal.pone.0147152. Accessed 18 Dec 2020.

Kutschera, Ulrich. 2018. *Das Gender-Paradoxon: Mann und Frau als evolvierte Menschentypen*. Münster: LIT Verlag.

Labisch, Alfons, and Reinhardt Spree, eds. 1989. *Medizinische Deutungsmacht im sozialen Wandel*. Bonn: Psychiatrie-Verlag.

Labisch, Alfons. 1991. Der öffentliche Gesundheitsdienst (öGD) angesichts neuer öffentlicher Gesundheitsleistungen ("new public health"). In *Oeffentliche Gesundheit - Public Health - Konzepte und Diskussionen in der deutschen Geschichte*, 84–102. Frankfurt a. M.: Campus.

LaFrance, Adrienne. 2020. The Prophecies of Q. American Conspiracy Theories Are Entering a Dangerous New Phase. *The Atlantic* (online). https://www.theatlantic.com/magazine/archive/2020/06/qanon-nothing-can-stop-what-is-coming/610567/. Accessed 30 Dec 2020.

Lamb, Vanessa. 2018. Who Knows the River? Gender, Expertise, and the Politics of Local Ecological Knowledge Production of the Salween River, Thai-Myanmar Border. *Gender, Place & Culture* 25 (12): 1703–1718.

Landesman, Robert, Robert E. Kaye, and Kathleen H. Wilson. 1973. Menstrual Extraction: Review of 400 Procedures at the Women's Services, New York, New York. *Contraception* 8 (6): 527–539. https://doi.org/10.1016/0010-7824(73)90095-4. Accessed 18 Dec 2020.

Langford-Hall, Mary. 2016. Recruitment, Retention and Mentoring of Minorities into the Fields of Communication Sciences and Disorders. *International Journal of Humanities and Social Science Review* 2 (9): 1–4.

Latour, Bruno. 2002. *Die Hoffnung der Pandora: Untersuchungen zur Wirklichkeit der Wissenschaft*. Frankfurt a. M: Suhrkamp.

Lee, Timothy B. 2015. *Ben Carson: The Ark was Built by Amateurs, the Titanic by Professionals.* *Vox.* https://www.vox.com/policy-and-politics/2015/10/29/9639228/ben-carson-noahs-ark. Accessed 25 July 2021.

Leonhard, Nina, and Astrid Mignon Kirchhof. 2015. Einführung: Gegenwelten. *Geschichte und Gesellschaft* 41: 5–16.

Lepore, Jill. 2015. *The Secret History of Wonder Woman.* First Vintage Books ed. New York: Vintage Books, A Division of Random House LLC.

Lewis, Tania. 2006. DIY Selves? Reflexivity and Habitus in Young People's Use of the Internet for Health Information. *European Journal of Cultural Studies* 9 (4): 461–479.

Lewis, Helen. 2020. The Coronavirus Is a Disaster for Feminism. Pandemics Affect Men and Women Differently. *The Atlantic* (online). https://www.theatlantic.com/international/archive/2020/03/feminism-womens-rights-coronavirus-covid19/608302/. Accessed 18 Dec 2020.

Linek, Jenny, and Pierre Pfütsch. 2016. Geschlechterbilder in der Gesundheitsaufklärung im deutsch-deutschen Vergleich (1949–1990). *Medizin, Gesellschaft und Geschichte* 34: 73–110.

Lippman, Abby, Anne Rochon Ford, and Kathleen O'Grady. 2008. Barbara Seaman (1935–2008): Pioneer in the Women's Health Movement. *Network Magazine of the Canadian Women's Health Network* 10 (2): 18–19.

Longino, Helen. 1990. *Science as Social Knowledge: Values and Objectivity in Scientific Inquiry.* Princeton: Princeton University Press.

———. 1994. In Search of Feminist Epistemology. *The Monist* 77 (4): 472–458.

———. 1995. Gender, Politics, and the Theoretical Virtues. *Synthese* 104 (3): 383–397.

———. 1997. Feminist Epistemology as Local Epistemology. *Proceedings of the Aristotelian Society, Supplementary Volumes* 71: 19–35, & 37–54.

Los Angeles Womens Center. 1973. *Sister: Self-Help Health Care 4.* Los Angeles.

LRA. Living River Association. 2020. *Training and Enhancing the Thai Baan Research Network. Both Domestic and International.* http://www.livingriver-siam.org/our-work?view=article&id=32:tbr-training&catid=32:taibaan. Accessed 18 Dec 2020.

Lupton, Deborah. 1995. *Medicine as Culture. Illness, Disease and the Body in Western Societies.* London/Thousand Oaks/New Delhi: Sage.

———. 2014. The Commodification of Patient Opinion: The Digital Patient Experience Economy in the Age of Big Data. *Sociology of Health & Illness* 36 (6). https://doi.org/10.1111/1467-9566.12109. Accessed 18 Dec 2020.

Magnezi, Racheli, Yoav S. Bergman, and Dafna Grosberg. 2014. Online Activity and Participation in Treatment Affects the Perceived Efficacy of Social Health

Networks Among Patients with Chronic Illness. *Journal of Medical Internet Research* 16 (1). https://doi.org/10.2196/jmir.2630. Accessed 18 Dec 2020.

Magubane, Zine. 2014. Spectacles and Scholarship: Caster Semenya, Intersex Studies, and the Problem of Race in Feminist Theory. *Journal of Women in Culture and Society* 39 (3). https://doi.org/10.1086/674301.

Mahr, Dana. 2017. Self-Reporting and Participatory Health Platforms: Empowerment Through Sharing Information About Oneself Online? *Harvard Bill of Health*. https://blog.petrieflom.law.harvard.edu/2017/05/01/self-reporting-and-participatory-health-platforms-empowerment-through-sharing-information-about-oneself-online/. Accessed 18 Dec 2020.

———. 2019. Mikrobiomisches Empowerment. Sind DIY Stuhltransplantationen Ein Weg Zu Mehr Gesundheitspraktischer Selbstwirksamkeit Für PatientInnen Mit Chronischen Darmerkrankungen. In *Personal Health Science*, ed. Nils B. Heyen, Sascha Dickel, and Anne Brüninghaus, 43–66. Munich: Springer.

Mahr, Dana, and Sascha Dickel. 2019. Citizen Science Beyond Invited Participation: Nineteenth Century Amateur Naturalists, Epistemic Autonomy, and Big Data Approaches Avant La Lettre. *History and Philosophy of the Life Sciences* 41 (4). https://doi.org/10.1007/s40656-019-0280-z. Accessed 18 Dec 2020.

———. 2020. Rethinking Intellectual Property Rights and Commons-Based Peer Production in Times of Crisis: The Case of COVID-19 and 3D Printed Medical Devices. *Journal of Intellectual Property Law & Practice* 15 (9): 711–717.

Mahr, Dana, and Livia Prüll. 2018. Körperliche Selbstermächtigung aus dem 3D-Drucker? Feministische Kulturen als Parallelwelten und der Kampf um gesellschaftliche Teilhabe seit 1970. In *Kybernetik, Kapitalismus, Revolutionen. Emanzipatorische Perspektiven im technologischen Wandel*, ed. Paul Buckermann, Anne Koppenburg, and Simon Schaub, 161–190. Münster: Unrast.

Mahr, Dana, Claudia Göbel, Alan Irwin, and Katrin Vohland. 2018. Watching or Being Watched – Enhancing Productive Discussion Between the Citizen Sciences, the Social Sciences and the Humanities. In *Citizen Science: Innovation in Open Science, Society and Policy*, ed. Susanne Hecker, Muki Haklay, Anne Bowser, Zen Makuch, and Johannes Vogel. London: UCL Press. https://doi.org/10.14324.

Mahr, Dana, Eva Mahr, and Christoph Rehmann-Sutter. 2019. Subjektivierungsfiguren Genetischer Information. *Sozialer Sinn* 20 (1): 1–39. https://doi.org/10.1515/sosi-2019-0001. Accessed 18 Dec 2020.

Mahr, Dana, Eva Mahr, and Martina Von Arx. 2019. *Entgrenzte Forschung. Soziologische und wissenshistorische Argumente Für eine Multiperspektivische Und kontextsensitive Regulierung von Risiken in der Humanforschung.* https://www.bag.admin.ch/bag/en/home/das-bag/ressortforschung-evaluation/forschung-im-bag/forschung-biomedizin/ressortforschungsprojekte-humanforschung.html#-658046932. Accessed 18 Dec 2020.

Marieskind, Helen I., and Barbara Ehrenreich. 1975. Toward Socialist Medicine: The Women's Health Movement. *Social Policy* 6 (2): 34–42.

Marshall, Eliot. 1987. Tobacco Science Wars; the Industry Has Been Bullying Scientists, According to Researchers Who Lead the Campaign Against Environmental Tobacco Smoke. *Science* 236: 250p.

Martinez, Bibiana, Francis Dailey, Christopher V. Almario, Michelle S. Keller, Mansee Desai, Taylor Dupuy, Sasan Mosadeghi, Cynthia Whitman, Karen Lasch, Lyann Ursos, and Brennan M.R. Spiegel. 2017. Patient Understanding of the Risks and Benefits of Biologic Therapies in Inflammatory Bowel Disease: Insights from a Large-Scale Analysis of Social Media Platforms. *Inflammatory Bowel Diseases* 23 (7): 1057–1064.

Missingham, Bruce D. 2003a. *The Environmental Evaluation on Social and Economic Conditions of the Population Receiving Impact on Housing: Pak Man Hydropower Project.* Final Report. http://mrcmekong.org/assets/Consultations/LuangPrabang-Hydropower-Project/LPHPP_PNPCA-Report_Vol-4-Part-1-of-3Marked.pdf. Accessed 18 Dec 2020.

———. 2003b. Forging Solidarity and Identity in the Assembly of the Poor. From Local Struggle to National Social Movement in Thailand. *Asian Studies Review* 27 (3): 317–340.

Möbius, Paul Julius, and Carmen de Burgos. 1900. *La inferioridad mental la mujer: (la deficiencia mental fisiologica de la mujer).* F. Sempere y Cia.

Molle, Francois, Tira Foran, and Mira Käkönen, eds. 2009. *Contested Waterscapes in the Mekong Region. Hydropower, Livelihoods and Governance.* London: Earthscan.

Moran, Rachel Louise. 2018. *Governing Bodies. American Politics and the Shaping of the Modern Physique.* Philadelphia: University of Pennsylvania Press.

Morgen, Sandra. 2002. *Into Our Own Hands: The Women's Health Movement in the United States, 1969–1990.* New Brunswick: Rutgers University Press.

Moscucci, Ornella. 1990. *The Science of Women: Gynaecology and Gender in England, 1800–1929.* Cambridge: Cambridge University Press.

Mosse, George L. 1990. *Die Geschichte des Rassismus in Europa.* Frankfurt a. M.: Suhrkamp.

Mulligan, Lesa Jean. 1983. Some Effects of the Women's Health Movement. *Topics in Clinical Nursing* 4 (4): 1–9.

Myint, Tun. 2016. *Citizen Science in a Democracy: The Case of Thai Baan Research.* Tocquevill Lecture. https://ostromworkshop.indiana.edu/pdf/seriespapers/2016F_Tocq/Myint%20paper.pdf. Accessed 25 July 2021.

National Research Council (US). 2011. *Committee on A Framework for Developing a New Taxonomy of Disease. Toward Precision Medicine: Building a Knowledge Network for Biomedical Research and a New Taxonomy of Disease. The National Academies Collection: Reports Funded by National Institutes of Health.* Washington, DC: National Academies Press. http://www.ncbi.nlm.nih.gov/books/NBK91503/. Accessed 18 Dec 2020.

Nature. editorial board. anonymous. 2020. Science Benefits from Diversity. Improving he Participation of Under – Represented Groups Is Not Just Fairer – It Could Produce Better Research. *Nature* 558. https://www.nature.com/articles/d41586-018-05326-3. Accessed 18 Dec 2020.

Neal, Lisa, Gitte Lindgaard, Kate Oakley, Derek Hansen, Sandra Kogan, Jan Marco Leimeister, Ted Selker. 2006. "Online Health Communities" 'CHI' 06. *Extended Abstracts on Human Factors in Computing Systems,* 444–447. New York: Association for Computing Machinery. https://doi.org/10.1145/1125451.1125549. Accessed 18 Dec 2020.

Nelson, Alondra. 2011. *Body and Soul. The Black Panther Party and the Fight Against Medical Discrimination.* Minneapolis: University of Minnesota Press.

Nelson, Jennifer. 2015. *More than Medicine: A History of the Feminist Women's Health Movement.* New York: New York University Press.

Nelson, Nici, and Susan Wright, eds. 1995. *Power and Participatory Development. Theory and practice.* Exeter: Intermediate Technology Publications.

Nichols, Francis H. 2000. History of the Women's Health Movement in the 20th Century. *Journal of Obstetric, Gynecologic, and Neonatal Nursing* 29 (1): 56–64.

Nikolow, Sybilla, and Arne Schirrmacher, eds. 2007. *Wissenschaft und Oeffentlichkeit als Ressourcen füreinander. Studien zur Wissenschaftsgeschichte im 20. Jahrhundert.* Frankfurt a. M.: Campus.

O'Neil, Cathy. 2016. *Weapons of Math Destruction. How Big Data Increases Inequality and Threatens Democracy.* London: Penguin Books.

OpenSNP. 2020. *FAQ.* https://opensnp.org/faq. Accessed 18 Dec 2020.

Oudshoorn, Nelly. 2001. On Bodies, Technology and Feminism. In *Feminism in Twentieth Century Science, Technology and Medicine,* ed. Angela N.H. Creager, Elizabeth Lunbeck, and Londa Schiebinger, 199–213. Chicago/London: University of Chicago Press.

Pasquale, Frank. 2015. *The Black Box Society: The Secret Algorithms That Control Money and Information.* Cambridge/London: Harvard University Press.

PatiensLikeMe blog. 2011. *Openness Philosophy.* http://blog.patients-likeme.com/2011/02/22/patient-choices-the-shape-of-sharing/. Accessed 18 Dec 2020.

PatientsLikeme. 2014. *Data for Good.* https://www.facebook.com/PatientsLikeMe/posts/10152402576804177. Accessed 18 Dec 2020.

———. 2016. *Blog: Data for Good.* https://blog.patientslikeme.com/a-new-year-a-new-goal/. Accessed 25 July 2021.

———. 2020. *Overview PLM.* https://www.patientslikeme.com/. Accessed 18 Dec 2020.

Paxton, Ken. 2020. *Health Care Professionals and Facilities, Including Abortion Providers, Must Immediately Stop All Medically Unnecessary Surgeries and Procedures to Preserve Resources to Fight COVID-19 Pandemic.* https://www.texasattorneygeneral.gov/news/releases/health-care-professionals-and-facilities-including-abortion-providers-must-immediately-stop-all. Accessed 18 Dec 2020.

Peuckert, Detlev. 1987. *Die Weimarer Republik: Krisenjahre der Klassischen Moderne.* Frankfurt a. M.: Suhrkamp.

Planert, Ute. 2000. Der dreifache Körper des Volkes: Sexualität, Biopolitik und die Wissenschaften vom Leben. *Geschichte und Gesellschaft* 26: 539–576.

Pomun, Teerapong. 2010. *Local Knowledge and Food Security in the Mekong River Basin.* http://www.livingriversiam.org/2work/tb/tb_a8.pdf. Accessed 18 Dec 2020.

Porter, Theodore M. 1995. *Trust in Numbers. The Pursuit of Objectivity in Science and Public Life.* Princeton: Princeton University Press.

Prainsack, Barbara. 2013. Let's Get Real About Virtual. Online Health Is Here to Stay. *Genetics Research* 95 (4). https://doi.org/10.1017/S001667231300013X. Accessed 18 Dec 2020.

———. 2014. The Powers of Participatory Medicine. *PLoS Biology* 12 (4): e1001837. Accessed 18 Dec 2020.

———. 2020. Data Mining in Systems Medicine and the Project of Solidarity: The Interface of Genomics and Society Revisited. In *De-Sequencing. Identity Work with Genes*, ed. Dana Mahr and Martina von Arx, 97–117. Basingstoke: Palgrave Macmillan.

Prainsack, Barbara, and Alena Buyx. 2017. *Solidarity in Biomedicine and Beyond.* Cambridge: Cambridge University Press.

Prüll, Livia. 2016. *Trans* im Glück. Geschlechtsangleichung als Chance. Autobiographie, Medizingeschichte, Medizinethik.* Göttingen: Vandenhoeck & Ruprecht.

Prüll, Cay-Rüdiger (now Livia Prüll). 2013. Making Sense of Diabetes: Public Discussions in early West Germany 1945 to 1970. In *Making Sense as a Cultural Practice*, ed. Jörg Rogge, 225–239. Bielefeld: Transcript.

reddit. 2017. *R/CrohnsDisease*. https://www.reddit.com/r/CrohnsDisease/. Accessed 18 Dec 2020.

———. 2020. *R/CrohnsDisease*. https://www.reddit.com/r/CrohnsDisease/. Accessed 18 Dec 2020.

Reddit r/IAmA. 2012. *Crohn's Experience*. https://www.reddit.com/r/IAmA/. Accessed 25 July 2021.

Rippon, Gina. 2019. *The Gendered Brain. The New Neuroscience that Shatters the Myth of the Female Brain*. London: Vintage Publishing.

Rochelle, Tina L., and Helen Fidler. 2012. The Importance of Illness Perceptions, Quality of Life and Psychological Status in Patients with Ulcerative Colitis and Crohn's Disease. *Journal of Health Psychology* 18 (7): 972–983.

Roe v. Wade. 410 U.S. 113. 1973. Braveman, Paula. 2010. Social Conditions, Health Equity, and Human Rights. *Health Hum Rights* 12 (2): 31–48. PMID: 21178188.

Roukos, Dimitrios H. 2012. Longevity with Systems Medicine? Epigenome, Genome and Environment Interactions Network. *Epigenomics* 4 (2): 119–123.

Rubino, Michael. 2015. The Boy with Half a Brain. *Indianapolis Monthly*, December 23. https://www.indianapolismonthly.com/longform/boy-with-half-brain-william-buttars. Accessed 18 Dec 2020.

Ruzek, Sheryl Burt. 1978. *The Women's Health Movement: Feminist Alternatives to Medical Control*. New York: Praeger.

Sammer, Christian. 2015. Die "Modernisierung" der Gesundheitsaufklärung in beiden deutschen Staaten zwischen 1949 und 1975. *Medizinhistorisches Journal* 50: 249–294.

Seaman, Barbara. 1995 (=1975). *The Doctor's Case Against the Pill*. 25th anniversary ed. Alameda and Emeryville Hunter House, Publishers Group West.

Shapin, Steven. 2010. *Never Pure. Historical Studies of Science as if It Was Produced by People with Bodies, Situated in Time, Space, Culture, and Society, and Struggling for Credibility and Authority*. Baltimore: Johns Hopkins University Press.

Shapiro, Ben. 2019. *Facts Don't Care About Your Feelings*. Hermosa Beach: Creators Publishing.

Singer, Natasha. 2020. New Data Rules Could Empower Patients but Undermine Their Privacy. *The New York Times*, March 9. https://elemental.medium.com/biohackers-with-diabetes-are-making-their-own-insulin-edbfbea8386d. Accessed 18 Dec 2020.

Smith, Dana G. 2019. Biohackers with Diabetes Are Making Their Own Insulin. *Medium* (online). https://elemental.medium.com/biohackers-with-diabetes-are-making-their-own-insulin-edbfbea8386d. Accessed 18 Dec 2020.

Söderfeldt, Ylva. 2013. *From Pathology to Public Sphere. The German Deaf Movement 1848–1914*. Bielefeld: Transcript.

Span, Paula. 1980. A New Era for Feminist Health Clinics. *The New York Times*, November 23.

Star, Susan Leigh, and R. James. 1989. Institutional Ecology, "Translations" and Boundary Objects: Amateurs and Professionals in Berkeley's Museum of Vertebrate Zoology, 1907–39. *Social Studies of Science* 19 (3): 387–420.

Stern, Jessica. 2020. The Concept of "Safe Spaces" Under COVID-19. *womensnews.org*. https://womensenews.org/2020/05/the-concept-of-safe-spaces-under-covid-19/. Accessed 18 Dec 2020.

Stollberg, Gunnar. 2001. *Medizinsoziologie. Einsichten*, Themen der Soziologie. Bielefeld: Transcript.

Strasser, Bruno J, and Dana Mahr. 2017. Experiential Knowledge, Public Participation, and the Challenge to the Authority of Science in the 1970s. *Harvard Bill of Health*. https://blog.petrieflom.law.harvard.edu/2017/05/02/experiential-knowledge-public-participation-and-the-challenge-to-the-authority-of-science-in-the-1970s/. Accessed 18 Dec 2020.

Strasser, Bruno, Jerome Baudry, Dana Mahr, Gabriela Sanchez, and Elise Tancoigne. 2019. Citizen Science? Rethinking Science and Public Participation. *Science & Technology Studies* 32 (2): 52–76.

Stringer, Judy, M. Anderson, R.W. Beard, D.V. Fairweather, and S.J. Steele. 1975. Very Early Termination of Pregnancy (Menstrual Extraction). *BMJ* 3 (5974): 7–9. https://doi.org/10.1136/bmj.3.5974.7. Accessed 18 Dec 2020.

Stuckler, David, and Sanjay Basu. 2013. *The Body Economic. Why Austerity Kills*. New York: Basic Books.

Suwankhong, Dusanee, and Pranee Liamputtong. 2015. Cultural Insiders and Research Fieldwork: Case Examples from Cross-Cultural Research with Thai People. *International Journal of Qualitative Methods* 14 (5). https://doi.org/10.1177/2F1609406915621404. Accessed 18 Dec 2020.

Swiss Personalized Health Network (SPHN). 2020. *Infrastructure Building to Enable Nationwide Use and Exchange of Health Data for Research*. https://sphn.ch/. Accessed 25 July 2021.

Taubert, Marco, Arno Villringer, and Patrick Ragert. 2012. Learning-Related Gray and White Matter Changes in Humans: An Update. *The Neuroscientist* 18 (4): 320–325.

Tavernise, Sabrina. 2017. Ben Shapiro, a Provocative "Gladiator", Battles to Win Young Conservatives. *The New York Times* (online). https://www.nytimes.com/2017/11/23/us/ben-shapiro-conservative.html. Accessed 18 Dec 2020.

TelAbortion. 2020. *Safe. Effective. Private. Convenient.* https://telabortion.org/. Accessed 18 Dec 2020.

Tempini, Niccolo. 2014. PatientsLikeMe.com: Developing Medical Research from Social Data. *LSE Research Festival 2014*, 2014-05-08. http://eprints.lse.ac.uk/57927/. Accessed 18 Dec 2020.

Tempini, Niccolo, and Lorenzo del Savio. 2018. Digital Orphans: Data Closure and Openness in Patient-Powered Networks. *BioSocieties* 14: 205–227.

The Feminist Counselling Collective. 1975. Feminist Psychotherapy. *Social Policy* 6 (2): 54–62.

The Power of Poop. 2016. *The Power of Poop | Promoting Safe Accessible Fecal Transplant.* http://thepowerofpoop.com/. Accessed 18 Dec 2020.

Todd-Gher, Jaime, and Payal K. Shah. 2020. Abortion in the Context of COVID-19: A Human Rights Imperative. *Sexual and Reproductive Health Matters* 28 (1). https://doi.org/10.1080/26410397.2020.1758394.

Tsang, Mary. 2020. *Open Source Estrogen. Housewives Making Drugs.* https://www.media.mit.edu/projects/open-source-estrogen/overview/. Accessed 18 Dec 2020.

Uebel, Thomas. 2020. Vienna Circle. *Stanford Encyclopedia of Philosophy.* https://plato.stanford.edu/cgi-bin/encyclopedia/archinfo.cgi?entry=vienna-circle. Accessed 18 Dec 2020.

Uhlig, Anne C. 2012. *Ethnographie der Gehörlosen. Kultur – Kommunikation – Gemeinschaft.* Bielefeld: Transcript.

Verbrugge, Lois M. 1982. The Women's Health Movement: Feminist Alternatives to Medical Control. *Sex Roles* 8 (2): 222–224.

Viloria, Hida, and Maria Nieto. 2020. *The Spectrum of Sex. The Science of Male, Female, and Intersex.* London: Jessica Kingsley Publishers.

von Krafft-Ebing, Richard. 1890. *Lehrbuch der Psychiatrie. Auf klinischer Grundlage für praktische Ärzte und Studierende.* 4th ed. Stuttgart: Enke.

von Soden, Kristine. 1988. *Die Sexualberatungsstellen der Weimarer Republik 1919–1933.* Berlin: Edition Hentrich.

von Wahl, Angelika. 2019. From Object to Subject: Intersex Activism and the Rise and Fall of the Gender Binary in Germany, Social Politics. *International Studies in Gender, State & Society.* https://doi.org/10.1093/sp/jxz044. Accessed 18 Dec 2020.

Warren, Michael, Jamie Gangel, and Elizabeth Stuart. 2020. Jared Kushner Bragged in April that Trump Was Taking the Country 'Back from the

Doctors'. *CNN Politics*. https://edition.cnn.com/2020/10/28/politics/woodward-kushner-coronavirus-doctors/index.html. Accessed 18 Dec 2020.

Watanaputi, Chayan. 2010. *Thai Baan Research Community Research for Community.* http://www.livingriversiam.org/2work/tb/tb_a2.html. Accessed 18 Dec 2020.

Weinberger, David. 2012. *Too Big to Know: Rethinking Knowledge Now that the Facts Aren't the Facts, Experts Are Everywhere, and the Smartest Person in the Room Is the Room.* New York: Basic Books.

Weingart, Peter. 2001. *Die Stunde der Wahrheit. Zum Verhältnis der Wissenschaft zu Politik, Wirtschaft und Medien in der Wissensgesellschaft.* Weilerswist: Velbrück Verlag.

Wicks, Paul, Timothy E. Vaughan, Michael P. Massagli, and James Heywood. 2011. Accelerated Clinical Discovery Using Self-Reported Patient Data Collected Online and a Patient-Matching Algorithm. *Nature Biotechnology* 29 (5): 411–414. Accessed 18 Dec 2020.

Wide. Feminists transforming Economic Development. 2020. *Covid-19 Crisis from a Feminist Perspective.* https://wideplus.org/2020/03/26/covid-19-crisis-from-a-feminist-perspective-overview-of-different-articles-published/. Accessed 18 Dec 2020.

Wiener, Norbert. 1948. *Cybernetics: Or Control and Communication in the Animal and the Machine.* Paris: Hermanm & Cie.

Wilburn, Jeanette, James Twiss, Karen Kemp, and Stephen P. McKenna. 2017. A Qualitative Study of the Impact of Crohn's Disease from a Patient's Perspective. *Frontline Gastroenterology* 8 (1): 68–73. https://doi.org/10.1136/flgastro-2015-100678. Accessed 18 Dec 2020.

Wilhelm, Nadja, and Dana (geb. Dominik) Mahr, and Christoph Rehmann-Sutter. 2015. Stoma als Wende. *Bauchredner* 1: 8.

Willis, Erin, and Marla B. Royne. 2017. Online Health Communities and Chronic Dsiease Self-Management. *Health Communication* 32: 269–278.

Willmes, David. 2013. *Zur Legitimität ethischer und sozialer Werte in der Wissenschaft.* Dissertation Bielefeld. https://pub.uni-bielefeld.de/download/2631123/2631127/Willmes_2013_Zur_Legitimitat_ethischer_und_sozialer_Werte_in_der_Wissenschaft.pdf. Accessed 18 Dec 2020.

Wohlsen, Marcus. 2011. Biopunk Kitchen-Counter Scientists Hack the Software of Life. *New York: Current* (online). https://www.overdrive.com/search?q=ACF7EAFA-86D0-402C-BB5A-EDAD02D44D4C. Accessed 18 Dec 2020.

World Health Organization, WHO. 2015. *Sexual Health, Human Rights and the Law.* https://apps.who.int/iris/bitstream/handle/10665/

175556/9789241564984_eng.pdf;jsessionid=6B51047279C2B0DC7F3B 6D1E717DFA58?sequence=1. Accessed 18 Dec 2020.

———. 2020. Q&A: *Violence Against Women During COVID-19.* https://www. who.int/emergencies/diseases/novel-coronavirus-2019/question-and-answers-hub/q-a-detail/violence-against-women-during-covid-19?gclid=Cj0 KCQjwupD4BRD4ARIsABJMmZ-q4EN7Vp4nhEZf7wzAd_ VGpIiYzv8o_rAbVdkGzlWbvK4SZA37apgaAoeaEALw_wcB.   Accessed 18 Dec 2020.

Yancy, Clyde W. 2020. COVID-19 and African Americans. *JAMA* 323 (19): 1891–1892. https://doi.org/10.1001/jama.2020.6548. Accessed 18 Dec 2020.

Yom-Tov, Elad. 2016. *Crowdsourced Health: How What You Do on the Internet Will Improve Medicine.* Cambridge: MIT Press.

Young, Kenneth A. 2014. Of Poop and Parasites: Unethical FDA Overregulation. *Food & Drug Law Journal* 69: 555–563.